Patterns of Aging

Contributions to Human Development

Vol. 3

Series Editors
K. F. Riegel, Ann Arbor, Mich. and *H. Thomae,* Bonn

S. Karger · Basel · München · Paris · London · New York · Sydney

Patterns of Aging

Findings from the Bonn Longitudinal Study of Aging

Volume Editor
H. Thomae
Department of Psychology, University of Bonn, Bonn

12 figures and 51 tables, 1976

S. Karger · Basel · München · Paris · London · New York · Sydney

Contributions to Human Development

(Successor to 'Bibliotheca «Vita Humana»')

Vol. 1: *Thomae, H.* and *Endo, T.* (Bonn): The Adolescent and His Environment. Contributions to an Ecology of Teen-Age Behavior. VI + 110 p., 6 fig., 6 tab., 1974.
ISBN 3-8055-1651-7

Vol. 2: Dialectic. Humanistic Rationale for Behavior and Development. J. F. *Rychlak*, West Lafayette, Ind. (ed). XI + 159 p, 1 fig., 1976
ISBN 3-8055-2288-6

Cataloging in Publication

Patterns of aging: findings from the Bonn longitudinal study of aging
Volume editor, H. Thomae. Basel, New York, Karger, 1976
(Contributions to human development, v. 3)
1. Aging
I. Thomae, Hans, 1915-ed. II. Title, III.
Series
WI CO778S v. 3/WT 104 P316

ISBN 3-8055-2292-4

Prindet in Switzerland by Thür AG, Offsetdruck, Pratteln
ISBN 3-8055-2292-4

Contents

Preface

This is the first report on a longitudinal study of aging which was started in 1965 at Bonn University. 220 men and women, born 1890–1895 and 1900–1905, coming from different parts of Western Germany, were observed during a period of 7 to 8 years. Findings point to a very complex pattern of variables correlated to consistency and change of behavior in old age. Socio-economic status, education, health, and perceived life situation are involved in the structuring of the aging process to at least the same degree as calendar age. Therefore the findings demonstrate the relevance of a differential gerontology, which defines different patterns of aging and the variables correlated with these patterns.

The editor should like to thank to all those who contributed to this study. In the first instance he should like to thank our subjects, those men and women who participated in the study. Next to this he should like to thank his co-workers, those who are represented in this book as authors, but also those who were most decisive for the success of this study as interviewers and research psychologists like Dr. *Maria Renner,* Dr. *Ingrid Tismer-Puschner,* Dr. *H. G. Tismer,* Dr. *Ursula von Langermann* und *Erlenkamp,* Prof. Dr. *N. Erlemeier* (now at Münster/W.), the late Dr. *Manfred Schreiner.* We also should like to thank Dr. med. *Klesper* who joined our staff as a specialist for internal medicine and Prof. Dr. med. *Kessler* who provided a medical checkup at the last measurement point.

The study was supported by the Stiftung Volkswagenwerk from 1964–1969 and by the Deutsche Forschungsgemeinschaft from 1970–1975.

Finally the editor should like to thank Mrs. *Angleitner-Binns* for her revision of the English translation and Dr. A. *Angleitner* for his valuable editorial assistance.

Bonn, December 16, 1975

H. *Thomae*

Contr. hum. Dev., vol. 3, pp. 1–11 (Karger, Basel 1976)

I. Background and Aims of the Bonn Longitudinal Study of Aging

Hans Thomae

Interindividual Variability in Gerontological Research

Findings from the Bethesda Study

Some of the most important findings of research on aging point to 'very large individual differences in intellectual performance among older persons' (*Birren et al.,* 1972, p. 37) and to different 'life styles' as 'an individual's characteristic way of performing the various social roles he is allocated by or which are related to his position in society' (*Birren et al.,* 1972, p. 64). Several outstanding approaches to the study of aging resulted in categorizations of 'types' of 'styles' of aging rather than in generalizing statements regarding decline or consistency of performance or adjustment (*Reichard et al.,* 1962; *Neugarten,* 1971; *Williams and Wirths,* 1965; *Maas and Kuypers,* 1974). *Birren et al.* (1963b, p. 314) summarized their findings on the personality of 'healthy' elderly men by stating that 'in marked contradiction to the usual stereotypes of "rigidity" and of "second childhood" these individuals generally demonstrated mental flexibility and alertness. They continued to be constructive in their living; they were resourceful and optimistic. The group was not uniform, however. Some individuals showed maladaptive patterns of withdrawal and depression. Some showed evidence of mental decline.'

Although the sample of the Bethesda Study was highly selective, already the first measurement showed a high degree of interindividual variability in the performance and behavior of persons belonging to the same age group.

Normative Study of Aging and Interindividual Variation

Although the interests of the workers of the Duke Gerontological Study on Aging were focused more on 'normal aging' (*Palmore,* 1970, 1974a, b), one of the main findings of this large interdisciplinary project pointed to the 'wide variation in aging patterns' (*Palmore,* 1974, p. 290). The assessment of this interindividual variation in biological and psychological findings therefore became one of the most relevant topics in the second progress report of this study (*Palmore,* 1974a, b).

Biological and Social Correlates of Cognitive Functioning: References to Interindividual Aspects of Aging

A very high degree of interindividual variability of intellectual performance of elderly persons was also demonstrated by numerous cross-sectional studies. *Birren and Morrison* (1961), *Kuhlen* (1963), *Granick and Friedman* (1967), *Green* (1969), *Nehrcke* (1972), and *Rudinger* (1974) pointed to differences in mental decline between persons from different educational backgrounds. Due to the great impact of education, many cross-sectional findings on mental decline with increasing age are misleading. According to *Schaie* (1965) and *Baltes* (1968), they reflect different educational opportunities in cohorts, e. g., born between 1880 and 1910 on the one hand, and those born between 1930 and 1960 on the other hand.

Another variable which contributes to interindividual differences in the aging process is related to occupational situation. As early as 1947, *Vernon* reported that age differences in intellectual performance are smaller if mental abilities are trained on the job. *Wagner* (1960) compared the intellectual performance and personality of a younger and an older group (average 50.2 years) of business executives. The older group performed at least at an equal level, if not better, than the younger one. On the other hand, however, interindividual variability was much higher in the older than in the younger group.

The important contributions of education and occupational situation to psychological differences between members of the same cohort are related to the socioeconomic status. *Britton et al.* (1967) and *Rudinger* (1974) demonstrated that SES explains the variance in WAIS performance to a greater degree than age.

Among the other variables which are closely related to differences in cognitive functioning and adjustment, physical health may be the most decisive one. The Bethesda Study on aged men (*Birren et al.*, 1963a) demonstrated this in the same way as did *Klonoff and Kennedy* (1966), *Spieth* (1964), *Hulicka* (1967), *Lehr et al.* (1972), and *Rudinger* (1974). All these studies support *Spieth*'s (1964) thesis, according to which 'mental decline' is a variable dependent on increasing health problems rather than on age.

Furthermore, we may mention those findings which are related to the stimulating effects of the environment on the cognitive and emotional-affective status of the ill and/or handicapped aged persons (*Weinstock and Benett,* 1969; *Gottesman,* 1973). As the environments of aged persons differ in degree of stimulation, interindividual variability is also to be expected as a result of this ecological factor.

There is some evidence that heredity is related not only to survivorship but also to the maintenance of a higher level of cognitive functioning in old age (*Jarvik,* 1962).

Individual Variation regarding Personality and Adjustment

A higher degree of interindividual variability in psychological functioning in older age groups is found also in studies on personality and adjustment. Aside from the studies of *Reichard et al.* (1962) and *Williams and Wirths* (1965), we might point here to the many variables which are correlated to life satisfaction in old age (*Adams,* 1973; *Thomae,* 1974a, b) to demonstrate the high degree of differences in this global measure for persons of the same age. Finally, we may refer to discussions on disengagement theory which pointed to the impact of biological and social conditions on the degree of social interaction reported by elderly people and their degree of satisfaction with this state of social interaction (*Neugarten and Havighurst,* 1969, p. 145.) *Neugarten and Havighurst* (1969) raise the question whether variation in social conditions solves the problem of individual variation, i. e., why some individuals are more content than others who live in the same general setting. In this connection, they point to personality as a common denominator for the crucial moderator variables.

'In attempting to understand why one individual copes successfully with retirement and another does not, we shall have to pursue in much greater depth the ways in which the aged individuals relate their pasts with their presents, and how they interpret and integrate their lives into meaningful wholes' (*Neugarten and Havighurst,* 1969, p. 446; see also *Maas and Kuypers,* 1974).

Differential Gerontology: A New Frame of Reference for Studies on Aging

This is just a selection of the findings which brought a new orientation in psychological research on aging: instead of defining general 'norms' for consistency and change of cognitive functioning and personality adjustment from middle to old age, the gerontologist tries to predict which patterns of aging resulting from the biological, psychological, and social conditions as they existed in earlier periods of the life cycle will emerge in the transition into old age as well as during this age period. Furthermore, the role of personality variables in the process of aging has become more and more evident.

Unfortunately, these personality variables very often are studied in terms of stable, inherited constructs while the impact of conditioning histories, of socialization in childhood, adolescence and young as well as middle adulthood is evaluated very often in an unsatisfactory way. However, if we conceive development as the outcome of some only partially identified genetic factors and of learning, we have to expect an increasing interindividual variability with increasing age.

This interindividual variability is programed by hereditary factors as we know from studies on longevity (*Jarvik,* 1962; *Rose and Bell,* 1971) and it is determined by the individual learning histories increasing in variety from youth to middle and old age (*Birren et al.*, 1972, p. 64). From this point of view, the aim of the study of aging should not be defined primarily in terms of the definition of a 'normal' age 'curve' or in terms of an average sequence of growth and decline. This is even more true if we consider the distorting effects of cross-sectional as well as of longitudinal studies regarding statements on 'normative' aging on the one hand (*Schale,* 1965; *Baltes,* 1968; *Rudinger,* 1972a–c) and the great difficulties existing for the realization of sequential studies which include a broader range of age and social class groups as well as a broader range of variables covered by the study (*Thomae et al.*, 1973; *Rudinger,* (1972a–c). Especially longitudinal studies can be vindicated against their critics only if they are focused on differential aspects of aging rather than on normative aspects. They demonstrate interindividual variability in aging and some of the conditions of this variability. From this point of view, they are instruments of prediction as well as of control of certain 'styles', 'patterns' or 'ways' of aging.

The Bonn Longitudinal Study of Aging – an Approach to a Differential Gerontology

General Hypothesis and Global Strategy

The planning and design of the Bonn Longitudinal Study on Aging (BLSA) was determined to a great degree by the findings reported above, which point to the increasing interindividual variability of biological, social, and psychological processes in older age.

The general hypothesis for the design refers to the complex character of the conditions which determine this interindividual variability. Therefore, the design was orientated more along the lines of 'global' longitudinal studies of children and adolescents which were started by *Jones* (1958), *McFarlane* (1938) and others around 1930. A study of this kind requires the inclusion of a great number of variables, whereas studies which are focused on a limited number of hypotheses can concentrate on one to three variables (e. g., *Owens,* 1966). However, our preference for the more global type of a longitudinal study is not based only on the expectation that 'aging' is an extremely complex process which differs under various biological, social, biographical and person-specific conditions. The history of the great longitudinal studies which have been started in the United States in the late twenties or early thirties of this century shows that some of the most valuable results of these studies emerged from hypotheses or theories which became relevant many years after the studies were started. When the Child Guidance Study (*McFarlane,* 1938) began in 1928, nobody cared about 'coping styles' or 'central orientations'. *Bronson* (1966), however was able to analyze the data collected in that study from 1928 to 1942 in terms of these constructs which had become important aspects of developmental theory since the late fifties of this century. She also could order early childhood data from 1928 to 1936 along a dimension 'expressive-outgoing vs. reserved-withdrawn', defined by her in 1966, and correlate these data with interview data from the same subjects as adults (*Bronson,* 1967). The very detailed analysis of the interviews with the mothers of the children of the Guidance Study provided by *McFarlane* (1938) enabled *Honzik* (1967) to interpret her findings on early childhood environmental correlates of mental growth until 30 years in terms of constructs defined 35 years after the beginning of the Guidance Study.

The careful registration of observational data on the children of the Fels Longitudinal Study enabled *Moss and Kagan* (1964) to have these data rated approximately 30 years later and to correlate them with ratings of interviews with the same subjects when they were adults. In fact, the most important aspect of this study rests on the definition of these rating scales which reflect the status of psychology theory between 1945 and 1960 rather than that of 1928.

As we keep our records available for future analysis, we expect that they, too, will provide material for testing hypotheses which today are unknown. But we hope that this volume will also demonstrate that we tried very hard to plan the study in a way which offers data for different kinds of theories and approaches.

On the other hand, the study had to make several restrictions in order to become materialized. As we included a fairly extensive psychological testing program, we had to limit the medical program out of financial as well as psychological reasons. However, a general health rating of each subject was made at each measurement point by a specialist of internal medicine. Furthermore, all survivors at the last measurement point (1972) had the most important tests in the University Hospital for internal medicine.

A second limitation refers to the assessment of learning and social conditions preceding transition into old age: they could be assessed only by interviewing the subjects themselves. Therefore, our findings are related to the reported socialization history rather than to the 'real' one. Our findings will have to be checked by the few studies which exist so far related to longer age ranges (*Owens,* 1966; *Maas and Kuypers,* 1974; *Palmore,* 1974a, b).

On the other hand, it was decided to take time enough to assess the physical, psyhological, economic and social situation of the subjects as it was perceived at each of the measurement points. We tried to take regard of the time perspective of this situation. Therefore, at each of the measurement points we devoted one 3-hour interview to the assessment of 'present situation', one inter-

Table I. Weekly schedule for testing program BLSA

	Measurement point		
	I	II	III/IV
Monday	informal meeting between staff and subjects	informal meeting between staff and subjects	informal meeting between staff and subjects
Tuesday a.m.	interview on present life situation, social participation, SES, etc.; daily round	interview on present life situation, etc.; changes in social situation; main events during past year	identical with measurement point II
p.m.	medical examination	medical examination	medical examination
Wednesday a.m.	life history interview (childhood, adolescence, young adulthood; life situation in 1948, 1955 and 1965)	life history interview (esp. the years 1960–1965); interview on self-perception, perceived social competence, etc.	life history interview focused on the most relevant stages in life
p.m.	free	free	free
Thursday a.m.	testing procedures: WAIS, TAT, Z test (short form of Rorschach), Riegel Scales	Raven, PM, Rorschach, Rosenzweig, PFT, Rosenberg, Scales on self-concept, Goodenough test	WAIS, Rorschach, self-concept, Goodenough test
p.m.	tour to the Rhine or Ahr Valley, behavior ratings by the participating observer	identical with measurement point I	identical with measurement point I
Friday a.m.	interview on future time perspective, on expected living conditions including attitudes towards institutionalization; Mierke psychomotor-performance test; measurement of variables in writing pressure.	interview abbreviated on future time perspective, including Bergius-Schreiner schedule; Mierke; Pursuit Rotor; identical with measurement point I	interview on future time perspective identical with measurement point I

view (between 2 and 4 h) to that of the past, and a third one to the assessment of the future outlook. Each interview was tape-recorded and as the tapes are still available it will be possible to use our data for future evaluations and hypothesis testing in the same way as this has been done with the very extensive records of the longitudinal studies of children and adolescents in Berkeley (*Baumrind,* 1966; *Bronson,* 1967) and in Yellowsprings (*Moss and Kagan,* 1964).

The schedule of our procedures at each of the first four measurement points (table I) demonstrates that we assigned the major part of the week during which our subjects were available to interviews. This decision can be explained firstly by methodological preferences which can be traced in the Berkeley Studies (*Jones,* 1958) in the same way as in ours. In our case this decision can be further supported by theoretical considerations which were formulated in terms of a 'cognitive theory of personality' (*Thomae,* 1968a–d), or of aging (*Thomae,* 1970) which places special emphasis on the nature of behavior as a dependent variable of the situation as perceived by the individual. As our subjects were well motivated to cooperate in our study, their responses in the interviews can be regarded as rather valid cues to their perceptions of present, past, and future life situation. On the other hand, we applied intelligence and personality tests to get information as objective as possible on their psychological situation. As cognitive and motivational aspects of behavior are interrelated to each other in a very complex manner, it was decided to introduce as many variables as possible in order to be able to identify different patterns of aging and the cognitive, motivational, social, and biological correlates of these patterns. The design of the study was influenced by the author's experience gathered as psychological director of the German Longitudinal Study on Children (*Coerper et al.,* 1954; *Hagen and Thomae,* 1962) and by longitudinal studies on middle-aged white-collar employees (*Lehr and Thomae,* 1958), as well as on a sample of men and women born between 1885 and 1930 (*Lehr and Thomae*, 1965; *Lehr*, 1969). The final design was discussed with many colleagues from Bonn and other Universities.

Time Limits for the Measurement Points

According to the 'global' orientation, the time schedule for each year of measurement allowed a week for each subject. The *Volkswagen Foundation,* which supported the project between 1964 and 1969, made this arrangement possible. In the last year (measurement point V, 1972), when the funds came from the German Research Union *(Deutsche Forschungsgemeinschaft),* the schedule had to be reduced to 2.5 days, due to increasing difficulties in finding support for basic research in social gerontology in the Federal Republic of Germany. This reduction changed the master plan for the assessment of variables mainly with regard to interview procedures, but may also have influenced other measures.

Overview of the Variables which BLSA Tried to Measure

(a) One set of variables which was assessed is related to social conditions existing immediately before the interview. Aside from careful assessment of the socioeconomic situation, we used the interview schedules of the cross-national study on adjustment to retirement (*Havighurst et al.*, 1969) to assess the degree and quality of social participation of our subjects. This schedule was supplemented by inventories related to leisure time activities, etc.

(b) A second set of information to be gathered was related to the past. We collected data on the life history from childhood up to the time of marriage and/or end of training for a job and inquired systematically about the time during and after World War II, in which most of the 'younger' men (born between 1900 and 1905) had to participate as soldiers. Using the time of the West German currency reform in 1948 as a reference point, it was very easy to elicit very detailed reports on the situation as it existed at the time regarding income, job, housing conditions, health and family. The interviewers tried not only to cover the situation as it was experienced; they asked in a detailed way for descriptions of how our subjects coped with different aspects of the situation.

The same procedure was followed for the reference times 1955 (i. e. 10 years before the first interview), 1965, 1966, 1968, 1970, and 1972. These reference points in time made it possible for most subjects to remember a very stressful situation and the ways they coped with it. Our data on perceived stress during these years from 1948 to 1972 point to a continuous decrease, which resulted in a decrease of information regarding the ways to cope with problems. However, this whole section will deserve special attention in the future evaluation of our data.

(c) A third set of data was related to plans for the year following the interview and in the more distant future. From a complex set of items we tried to rate extension and quality of future time perspective, attitudes toward health and death, etc.

(d) Our test data included the HAWIE (German standardization of WAIS) at the first, third, fourth and fifth measurement point and the Raven Progressive Matrices in the 2nd and 5th year. These tests are used in most studies on aging, but tests for checking psychomotor performance at high speed are less frequently used. We applied the Mierke apparatus (or 'Kieler Determinationsgerät'), in which subjects have to react to irregular patterns of colored flashes and of sounds with increasing speed (chap. IV, p. 36). Two other tests to measure psychomotor adjustment were used only in the first, respectively, last years of the study: a Pursuit Rotor learning task and the Beck apparatus.

(e) Projective techniques, used especially during the first years, were Rorschach and Behn-Rorschach, and *Wilde's* Wunsch-Probe ('wish test').

(f) Since questionnaires adapted for aged persons from lower middle class were not available at the time of the beginning of our study, we used the Riegel inventories (*Riegel,* 1960) which had been developed with an aged population in northern Germany in the late fifties. They try to assess several aspects of attitudinal rigidity, dogmatism, attitudes toward present and future time.

(g) Data on health and standard medical data were recorded at each measurement point in a standardized situation. In the last year a half-day clinical checkup was added.

Sampling Procedures

Most longitudinal studies on aged persons use volunteers who are motivated by organizations or agencies (*Birren et al.*, 1963b, p. 7) or by their cooperative attitude toward friends, colleagues, or relatives who ask them to participate (snowball technique, *Busse et al.,* 1970, p. 4; see also *Stone and Norris,* 1966, p. 575).

We tried very hard to draw a random sample of the western part of West Germany (Ruhr area, Cologne, Bonn and suburbs, Frankfurt, Mannheim, Heidelberg) for our study. However, in the same way as many previous researchers, we faced many difficulties in doing so. Sampling procedures for a 2-hour interview are a completely different matter compared to a complex psychological and medical examination which requires travel to and attendance at a university institute for a whole week.

Therefore we completed our random sample with referrals from welfare organizations and industrial plants to whom we explained our aims and plans. We required that persons participating should be in good health and live in their own household. The subjects we included had to be able to travel to Bonn by train and stay in a small hotel near the institute or, for those in the Bonn area, reach the institute every day using public transportation. Another selection requirement was lower middle-class or (to a small percentage) middle middle-class status. We tried also to control the sample for religious background and place of birth (West Germany versus former German provinces which belong now to Russia, Poland, and Czechoslovakia). A detailed description of the original sample will be given by *Rudinger and Schmitz-Scherzer* (chap. II, p. 12).

A major decision had to be made regarding the age cohort. In order to analyze possible effects of retirement, one half (about 110) of our subjects (59 men, 51 women) were looking forward to retirement or had retired no more than 2 years before the first point of measurement. A second cohort consisted mainly of persons who had retired 3–12 years before our study started. This resulted in a design which included four groups of men and women of lower middle-class status: (1) men born between 1900 and 1905, (2) women born between 1900 and 1905, (3) men born between 1890 and 1895 and (4) women born between 1890 and 1895.

This design made it possible to combine longitudinal and cross-sectional comparisons. The two cohorts did not differ regarding SES, and health differences were confined to the group of older women at the beginning of the study. However, the biography of the older cohort during childhood, adolescence, and young adulthood was characterized by the experience of peace and security, although they very often reported great economic need and few opportunities for better education or occupational training. The adulthood of the older men was influenced by military service during World War I, whereas the older women very often either lost their first husband or fiancé in this war or were separated from their husband for years. Very often they reported of great economic difficulties and even starvation for this time.

Only very few of the 'younger' men were soldiers in World War I (for the last year). Most of them were adolescents during this war and had to work quite hard to help support their families. A time remembered by both groups in the same intense and negative manner was around 1930 when there was widespread unemployment in Germany.

During the time between 1933 and 1945, most of our older subjects did not favor the Hitler regime. One survived many years in a concentration camp; others belonged to Christian groups in the silent opposition, and only a few apparently were supporters of the regime. On the other hand, the group born between 1900 and 1905 included at least one member of the SS troup and several active party members as well as quite a few supporters of the regime. Most of the younger group were in the German Army in World War II and most of them reported their experiences as prisoners of war.

From these data a cross-sectional comparison of our cohorts is reasonable, although the main emphasis of our study was on the longitudinal analysis.

Longitudinal Samples of Aged Persons – 'Normative' or 'Elite' Groups

Considering the many deprivations, stresses, and personal losses reported by most of our subjects, they could be regarded as the 'survivors' of serious strains even at the first point of measurement. The men in particular were survivors in the true sense of the word. According to census data of the FRG (1961), 1890–1895 cohorts consisted of about 1 million men and 1.658 million women; the 1900–1905 cohorts included 2.076 million men and about 2.5 million women. These sex differences in survivorship are only partially explained by the two world wars. More recent calculations point to the decreasing life expectancy for men in the next 10 years (*Schwarz,* 1974) compared to a slowly increasing life expectancy of women. This difference is explained by some writers with references to the occupational situation of men as entailing more severe stress and other conditions conducive to coronary vascular disease in middle age.

Against this background our subjects might be defined as a biological 'elite' even if they have by no means attained the status of centenarians. Especially those who were able to come to us at all points of measurement from 1965 to 1972 may be regarded as examples of 'successful' aging. It will be discussed later in this book (p. 147) to what extent we can consider this successful pattern to be a normative one. Inasmuch as this pattern is defined by the ability to lead a fairly independent life, it certainly is more representative of the aged population as a whole than the subjects of studies whose data usually are reported in gerontological and especially geriatric journals or in reports of social welfare agencies.

Of all persons living in the FRG aged 65 or above, approximately 96–97% live in their own household. Within our sample at measurement point I, 3–4% of the men and women were living in a home for the aged.

Unfortunately the image of the deteriorated, helpless or at least dependent old person has been reinforced by many clinical experts generalizing unduly from their experiences with physically or mentally impaired patients. Even if samples like ours here are to be defined as an 'elite' group (although they belong mainly to lower SES), studying them can help in revising stereotypes that have emerged from experiences with physically and/or economically highly dependent persons. The reports on our findings published so far have been evaluated by many clinicians, social workers and the general public as a much needed counterbalance to negative stereotypes of aged persons. In this book our main emphasis is on the demonstration of different patterns of aging and the development of ways to evaluate, predict, and control them. Therefore, the image of aging we should like to reinforce is neither optimistic nor pessimistic; it is realistic, i. e. adapted to the highly complex and variable process of aging.

Contr. hum. Dev., vol. 3, pp. 12–19 (Karger, Basel 1976)

II. Sample and Methods

Georg Rudinger and Reinhard Schmitz-Scherzer

Description of Sample

The circumstances under which the sample for the Bonn Longitudinal Study of Aging (BLSA) was gathered are described by the project's initiator *Thomae* in chapter I (pp. 1–11). The reasoning behind the choice of the two cohorts also need not be repeated. It almost goes without saying that the BLSA sample has been subject to attrition processes over the first 7 years of investigation (1965/66, first measurement point, to 1972/1973, fifth measurement point). Table I illustrates this fact. It remains to be seen whether changes in the sample's overall sociodemographic composition (e. g. *Schmitz-Scherzer,* 1975c) or systematically distorted results for the various dependent variables under study (e. g. chap. III) occur as a result of the loss of these particular 'dropouts'. Of course, wherever possible, the attempt is made to capitalize on opportunities raised by the otherwise disadvantageous effects of having subjects drop out. Therefore, we shall systematically study the circumstances under which subjects do drop out in the survivor study (chap. X) and in the present chapter.

The original sample at the first point of measurement in 1965/66 included 222 persons divided into the two above mentioned cohorts 1900–1905 and 1890–1895. The younger cohort consisted of 114 persons and the older one of 108. Of the 114 younger subjects, 55 were women and 59 men and in the older cohort there were 49 women and 59 men (table I).

Information on the demographic structure and socioeconomic characteristics of our sample should help complete the picture. This information is supplied below by giving data from measurement sessions I (1965/66) to V (1972/73), which are presented in conjunction to highlight whatever systematic changes may have occurred within the sample. The corresponding data from a control sample which participated in testing at the fifth measurement point is added as a basis for comparison.

Table I. Number of BLSA participants and dropouts (in parentheses) at all five points of measurement from 1965/66 to 1972/73 and number of control group participants in 1972/73

	Measurement point					Control
	I	II	III	IV	V	
Younger cohort						
Men	59 (4)	55 (8)	47 (7)	40 (4)	36	13
Women	55 (5)	50 (2)	48 (10)	38 (7)	31	22
Sum	114 (9)	105 (10)	95 (17)	78 (11)	67	35
Older cohort						
Men	59 (7)	52 (3)	49 (10)	39 (11)	28	13
Women	49 (4)	45 (5)	40 (11)	29 (3)	26	13
Sum	108 (11)	97 (8)	89 (21)	68 (1)	54	26
Total	222 (20)	202 (18)	184 (38)	146 (2)	121	61

In 7 years the original sample was reduced by 101 persons (about 46%). The proportional representation of both sexes, however, remained more or less unchanged. In contrast to the BLSA sample, there were more women than men in the control sample. Of the control sample participants, 26 were men (42.6%) and 35 were women (57.4%).

The causes leading to the reduced sample size are of some interest in this context. All in all, 44 persons (19.8% of the original sample) passed away. 40 (18.0% of the original sample) were prevented from returning by reasons of health or by family obligations (e. g. caring for sick spouse). Hopeless scheduling difficulties hindered only a few participants from appearing at the most recent measurement session. 17 persons either gave no information on why they could not appear or were among those who took part in some but not all measurement sessions.

Grombach (1975) has shown that the processes leading to reduced sample size maintained a steady rate in this study with no major deviations between the measurement points. This holds for both the preceding and the following results.

Comparing subjects who dropped out and subjects of the same sex and cohort who did not, we find that the dropouts do not differ noticeably from either the original or the longitudinal sample. The control group differs from the BLSA samples in that it has slightly over 10% fewer men and about 10% more women than the BLSA sample at measurement point V.

Although a few differences between the control group and the BLSA sample at measurement point V do become evident in respect to the distribution of the sexes, the assumption that the samples are largely comparable is warranted. This is shown by a number of similar means and standard deviations over the entire period of investigation, to be reported below, and is further supported by the distributions of socioeconomic data which will be discussed in more detail later.

The original BLSA sample, the reduced longitudinal sample, and the control group are comparable in respect to *income.* Nearly all participants completed grade school (through and including 8th grade). The most numerous contingent are those who attained the 'mittlere Reife' (10th grade). Graduates of college prep courses ('Gymnasium') or institutes of higher education ('Fachschule' or university) are relatively few. Women more frequently report that their schooling ended with the 'mittlere Reife', and men more often attained a degree from an institute of higher education. The original, longitudinal, and control samples are all similar in this regard.

At the beginning of the BLSA in 1965/66, 43 men (36.4%) and 11 women (10.6%) were still *working.* Twelve more men and 3 more women were earning some extra money on the side in a job-like situation. At the most recent measurement point in 1972/73, 12 men of the entire longitudinal sample were still working, and 7 men and 1 woman were engaged in a job-like activity.

In all of the samples, most of the women were homemakers and had either had no other job training or had not been employed for years. White-collar workers, civil servants, and skilled workers are the most frequently encountered occupational groups in the original sample and, on the whole, in the longitudinal and control groups as well.

The majority of the subjects lived in *rented appartments,* but quite a few owned their own homes. The proportion of those living in homes for the aged did not exceed the figure 3.5–4.5% found in the population at large. Only the control group had a slightly higher percentage.

A further point of relative similarity between the BLSA samples and the control group is the size of the community in which the subjects reside. The majority live in towns or small cities with up to 50,000 citizens or in large cities with populations over 100,000.

Using the set of information obtained in the course of the investigation about monthly income, education, job training, occupational position before retirement, housing arrangements, and other life circumstances, it was possible to rate the socioeconomic status of the subjects on a five-point scale (1 = very low to 5 = very high). The combined estimates of socioeconomic status describe these samples as belonging to the lower middle class. Over two thirds of the participants were thus classified by those who carried out the ratings.

The *marital status* distribution is typical for the older generation. Most participants are married, especially the men. A greater number of women are single or widowed.

The psychological investigation was accompanied by a *medical examination* with the aid of an internist. On the basis of a physical examination and interviews, the physician rated the subject's *general health* on a five-point scale from 1 = excellent to 5 = very poor. The results show the participants to be in relatively good health, especially for their age, compared to the generally poor health status frequently encountered in the literature on gerontological studies.

As mentioned above, it is only possible to obtain precise information contrasting 'survivors' with 'dropouts' in the context of a longitudinal study. A first step toward this description concentrated on comparing the initial sample with the *bona fide* longitudinal sample of those who were tested at every single measurement session to see if the two differ in respect to socioeconomic characteristics. Generally speaking, this was not the case in our sample. Thus, the results obtained for the longitudinal sample could 'reasonably' be generalized to include the original sample. It must be remembered, however, that this overall comparability of the two BLSA subsamples in no way reduces the possibility of systematic differences between them in regard to the various dependent variables under study; that is, it is possible for something like a 'selection process' involving psychological variables to take place (chap. III, X).

Turning to the control group, we find that it too is sufficiently comparable to the longitudinal sample, although less so than the original sample. Still, the comparison of these two groups is of special interest because it can provide information on the existence of test wiseness (*Campbell and Stanley,* 1963).

Selection of Variables

In chapter I (p. 6) of this volume, *Thomae* gives an overview of the variables which the BLSA tried to measure. The variables can be classified under seven headings. These categories are listed below, and references to the chapters concerning them are given in parentheses.

(1) Social conditions immediately before the interview. Social involvement (chap. VII). Leisure activities (chap. IX). Social indicators of a more specific nature such as education, occupation, housing conditions, etc., which enter into nearly all analyses as independent variables.

(2) Information on the past; perceived life history.

(3) Outlook on the future. (Chapter VIII deals with a number of variables from the second and especially the third category).

(4) Data from standardized psychometric tests; developments in performance on intelligence and psychomotor tests are described in chapters III and IV.

(5) Data from projective methods.

(6) Riegel questionnaire (chap. VI).

(7) Health and standard medical data.

These data frequently appear as independent variables or as correlates of the variables under consideration.

Selected variables from all seven categories are investigated by *Grombach* in chapter V in respect to structural changes over time as revealed by factor analytic methods. A set of variables drawn from all seven areas are examined by *Lehr and Schmitz-Scherzer* in chapter X as to whether they differentiate between survivors and nonsurvivors.

The variables in this report have been selected according to a number of considerations already mentioned by *Thomae* in this book (chap. I) and others (*Thomae et al.*, 1973) as falling within the scope of the BLSA's global hypothesis. Some additional selection criteria resulted from more technical considerations. For example, it made sense to limit the analysis to those variables which were recorded regularly for all participating subjects at all 3, 4, or 5 points of measurement under relatively constant 'experimental' conditions. The relevance and necessity of this limitation have already been made clear by the information given in chapter I on the organizational difficulties and investigation procedures of the study.

Still another selection criterium was applied, namely the reliability of the variables. The complexities involved in attempting to ascertain change using measurements of questionable reliability are widely recognized (*Lord,* 1967; *Bereiter,* 1967; *Cronbach and Furby,* 1970, to name but a few). In an attempt to isolate evidence of actual change from random fluctuations, the BLSA authors utilize several methods with varying capacities and objectives in order to determine the reliability, structural invariance, and constant validity of the variables. Generalizability studies (*Cronbach et al.*, 1972) were computed by *Rudinger and Feger* (1970) for the individual measurement points to test the generalizability of the variable 'overall impression', a behavior rating, the universes of raters and scales. Analyses of variance were used in accordance with *Winer*'s (1971) proposals to estimate the reliability at each point of measurement of further information, namely the HAWIE (German WAIS standardization), the behavior rating (*Rudinger,* 1975), and some scales related to subjective life space (*Opgenoorth,* 1971). There are numerous other studies which we may consider relevant to the question of separating reliability and stability from change, although this is not necessarily their main topic. These are studies using analyses of variance (persons x variables x measurement points) in terms of generalizability designs developed by *Cronbach et al.* (1972; see also *Lindquist,* 1953, chap. 10) as well as certain factor analytic studies as long as they stick to the variable patterns in drawing comparisons over time. Studies of this sort could serve as the preliminary stages of more detailed analyses leading to the identification of differential trends in psychological development. Following an analysis of variance with 'persons x variables x time', it would pay to proceed with further analyses given the following conditions: a substantial 'persons x variables' component, and sufficient indications that person differences and a relatively small 'variables x time' component occur in conjunction (the 'variables x time' component, indicating change in the variables over time independent of the persons, amounts to undesirable variance). Preparatory computations of this sort for BLSA material have been carried out for the variables 'overall impression' (*Rudinger and Feger,* 1970; *Grombach,* 1975), HAWIE (*Rudinger,* 1971a), Riegel questionnaires (*Angleitner,* 1974b), and leisure variables (*Schmitz-Scherzer,* 1975a-c).

In addition, there are also some studies dealing with the question of factor invariance over time, which provide a foundation for further factor score analyses suggested by *Nesselroade* (1970) and *Nesselroade et al.* (1972). These factor analyses cover the HAWIE (*Rudinger,* 1971a,c, 1974, 1975), behavior rating (*Grombach,* 1975), Riegel questionnaires (*Angleitner,* 1974a), several variables related to outlook toward the future (*Schreiner,* 1971a, b), and the above mentioned aspects of the BLSA global hypothesis (*Thomae et al.*, 1973; *Grombach,* 1975; chapter V of this volume).

Another possibility for testing the stability of the recorded measurements over time consists of correlating the factor scores over the measurement points (*Nesselroade and Baltes,* 1973). Similarly, *Fisseni* (chap. VIII) interprets the average correlation of the repeated measurements as a sign of stability/reliability. However, in these direct correlations, information due to stability and reliability becomes confounded. For this reason, another correlational procedure designed to circumvent this confounding will be used more often. Our proposal makes use of the path analytic approach to the assessment of reliability over all measurement points and the measurement of stability between two measurement points at a time. *Heise* (1971) developed this procedure on the basis of *Coleman*'s (1968) work. In addition to the usual psychometric assumptions it is also assumed that the reliability of the measured scores is stable over time.

Wiley and Wiley (1971) argue very convincingly that this additional assumption is a restrictive and doubtful one. The reliabilities and stabilities reported here should therefore be understood as tentative values which could be strengthened by a larger number of measurement points in the framework of *Heise*'s (1971) model or by application of the modified model of *Wiley and Wiley* (1971). The calculated reliabilities of the variables will not be listed here as they can be found in chapters V–VII and IX.

At this point we must once again point out the particular difficulty of establishing reliability when measuring change. The above mentioned methods for assessing reliability are all based on a trait conception. That is, they assume a relatively constant value of the variable in question over a period of time. As a result, change-resistant measurement instruments are sought and change-sensitive methods are disqualified as not reliable enough. In the present study, attention has repeatedly been drawn to the situational aspects of observed characteristics. Here the effort to assess change takes priority, and stability in the sense of reliability is hardly to be expected, or must at least be questioned. For these reasons, the reliability coefficients presented here must, as we have repeatedly pointed out, be seen in the context of the problematic reliability/true change relation.

Statistical Procedures

The research reports in this volume are addressed to the task of tracking down the conditions, 'causes', and determinants of differential processes in aging. This means working out differential patterns of aging in terms of various 'independent' dimensions of the variables under study. The majority of efforts reported in this book are aimed at finding these patterns of aging by comparisons of the observed measures of central tendency (mean or median) along the time dimension of longitudinal testing. Of course, each author introduces individual variations into this general approach, creating something like residual variance which transcends the explanatory range of the initial general statement.

In order to make inference statistical evaluations and comparisons possible in their examinations of quantitative changes over time, a number of contributors *(Rudinger, Grombach, Angleitner, Schmitz-Scherzer,* and *Lehr and Schmitz-Scherzer)* utilize an analysis of variance model with two or three factors and a repeated factor (time) (*Winer,* 1971). *Schmitz-Scherzer and Angleitner* computed analyses of covariance with intelligence, health and/or socioeconomic status as covariates: *Lehr and Schmitz-Scherzer* make use of analyses of covariance in comparing 'survivors' and 'nonsurvivors'. A glance at recent issues of the *Psychological Bulletin* shows that discussion about this delicate instrument (*Elashoff,* 1969) is still continuing.

In this collection of studies, widespread use is made of cohort groupings with the two cohorts described earlier, social characteristics (education, occupation, etc.), sex, and health (objective and subjective) as independent variables. Two additional variables, 'contentment with present situation' and 'extent of plans', are used as independent variables by *Grombach.*

Other attempts of comparisons of central tendency measures are based on t tests *(Lehr and Schmitz-Scherzer),* multiple t tests *(Mathey),* and nonparametric methods *(Olbrich and Lehr).*

The fond hopes expressed by *Schaie* (1970; *Schaie and Gribbin,* 1975) that data be revamped, so that other investigations can be carried out using sequential strategies, seem entirely plausible for BLSA material. By adding independent control groups from a separate gerontological study in 1968 and drawing up a BLSA control group in 1972 (see the description of the sample), it was possible to carry out both cross-sequential and time-sequential analyses as in the model of *Schaie* (1965, 1970, 1973; *Baltes,* 1968; *Baltes and Schaie,* 1973a, b; *Buss,* 1973, 1975; *Labouvie,* 1975; *Schaie and Baltes,* 1975).

The research concepts discussed so far fall under the heading of efforts to discover differential age patterns on the basis of classical external criteria such as age, cohort/generation, education, etc. Another approach is to draw up groups solely on the basis of directed change in the characteristics under study. Using the 'Konfigurationsfrequenzanalyse' method developed by *Lienert and Krauth* (1975), *Fisseni* undertakes to partition the sample into exclusive groups with characteristic patterns in respect to given variables. *Mathey* conducts part of his investigations by concentrating on subjects whose psychomotoric achievements either constantly improved or deteriorated over all five measurement points. Thus we might say that he selects the most extreme of all possible change patterns. It should be obvious that all the previously mentioned difficulties of interpreting observed variations as true change or measurement artifacts are still with us, even when the alternative research strategy finds application (*Lord,* 1967; *Bereiter,* 1967; *Cronbach and Furby,* 1970; *Furby,* 1973).

In addition to looking for quantitative changes, an interest in the investigation of structural changes has come to play an important role recently (*Bentler,* 1973; *Baltes and Nesselroade,* 1970, 1973; *Nesselroade,* 1970, 1972, 1973; *Buss,* 1974a–c, 1975). Except in the articles by *Grombach* and *Rudinger,* the latter consideration remains on the sidelines in most sections of the present publication. Yet there are several publications from the BLSA that have addressed themselves to investigating structural change (e. g. *Thomae et al.,* 1973). Such factor analytic results, however, are presently treated as the background for the evaluation of quantitative changes. *Grombach,* for example, organizes the treatment of his variables around his factor analysis. In the type of more extensive analyses which are called for, the persons would receive characteristic values on each factorial dimension, i. e. factor scores would become dependent variables (*Nesselroade et al.,* 1972). So far, such analyses have been incorporated into the BLSA only for the two HAWIE factors (handling of verbal material and perceptual and spatial organization), in connection with the pursuit of sequential strategies (*Rudinger,* 1973a, b). They will not be described here (*Rudinger and Schmitz-Scherzer,* 1976).

Contr. hum. Dev., vol. 3, pp. 20–35 (Karger, Basel 1976)

III. Correlates of Changes in Cognitive Functioning

Georg Rudinger

Introduction

The main purpose of the Bonn Longitudinal Study of Aging (BLSA) is the description and explication of ontogenetic interindividual variability and of interindividual differences in intraindividual variability (chap. I; *Rudinger,* 1975). There are some tentative answers to this central question in the BLSA, also for the area of cognitive performance in old age; preliminary work is done by cross-sectional studies of structure and determinants of intellectual functioning (*Rudinger,* 1971a–c) which pointed to the impact of age, health, education, occupation and sex, confirming many findings from US and European gerontological studies (*Baltes and Labouvie,* 1973; *Birren et al.,* 1963a, b; *Chown and Heron,* 1965; *Granick and Friedman,* 1967; *Jarvik et al.,* 1973; *Lehr,* 1972; *Loewe,* 1970; *Welford,* 1966; see also chapters I and XII, pp. xxx, of this volume). In this paper we want to report only on the longitudinal analysis which exists for time intervals of 3 years (first to third measurement point, MP, and second to fourth MP), 5 years (first to fourth MP) and 7 years (first to fifth MP). The larger the time span, the smaller the longitudinal sample, due to some well-known attrition processes (chap. II). For the time intervals of 3 and 5 years we could apply some sequential strategies according to the Schaie model. The dependent variables in these and the other analyses were in each case indices of cognitive intellectual functioning such as the verbal score (VS), performance score (PS) and full scale score (FS) of the 'Hamburg-Wechsler-Intelligenz-Test für Erwachsene' (HAWIE, the German equivalent of WAIS), or total scores of the Raven colored progressive matrices (CPM).

Results

As outlined in chapter II, we apply two designs in this section.

Design 1: The 'classical' variance analysis for repeated measurements (case II; *Winer,* 1971) each with three factors: (a) 'age' group/cohort, according to the initial arrangement, with two levels; (b) sex or educational level (three levels: high, medium, low) or socioeconomic status (SES; two levels), and (c) MPs with three levels for a sample n = 147, and four levels for a longitudinal sample n = 104. With this design we have the opportunity to find out whether different changes happened within a period of 5 or 7 years in the diverse groups defined in terms of several criteria such as age/cohort and sociocultural conditions.

Design 2: Sequential methods; cross-sequential (XS) analysis for the (dependent) longitudinal samples of BLSA and time-sequential (TS) analysis with controls drawn independently in 1968 and 1972 (chap. II).

The interactions 'age/cohort x time', 'sex x time', 'sociocultural aspects (education, SES) x time' within design 1 may comprehend important information because they indicate whether (a) there are age/cohort-specific developmental patterns in both parts of HAWIE; (b) there are different developmental patterns for men and women, on the background once more of the disuse-hypothesis or derived from studies of samples with different initial performance levels (*Terman and Oden,* 1959; *Tuddenham et al.,* 1968); probably of this kind that men maintain or even improve their performance and/or women drop below their poorer performance, and (c) in this short time period of 5 or 7 years there are certain trends of differential changes for groups with different initial intellectual levels operationalized by educational/occupational or (more global) by SES levels; at this point at the latest we enter the *inter*dependent interactionistic network of intelligence-education-occupation-stimulating life conditions – SES, etc. (*Birren and Woodruff,* 1973; *Kuhlen,* 1963; *Lehr,* 1972; *Loewe,* 1970; *Lorge,* 1936; *Rudinger,* 1974; *Schoenfeldt,* 1973), with a unidirectional design which allows only tentative, very restricted answers.

Thus we asked (1) for differences between groups and (2) for changes (time standing for the aging process) within different groups or for differences between changes within the groups. However, it should be reemphasized that these designs cannot be directly considered as pure sequential strategies.

As pointed out in chapter I by *Thomae* and in the introduction of the present chapter, a withdrawal from the concept of general intelligence and general decline with age has taken place in the history of psychogerontology in favor of a differential view, even with regard to the Wechsler test system (e. g. hold versus don't hold tests, etc., *Wechsler,* 1964). But a more formal and developmentally oriented model has been conceptualized in the context of fluid and crystallized intelligence (*Cattell,* 1963; *Horn and Cattell,* 1966, 1967).

The distinction between fluid and crystallized intelligence has the appeal of being an intrinsic part of a developmental concept of intelligence. Fluid intelligence is assumed to exhibit a pattern that closely matches the growth and decline of maturational and/or biological processes, that is, a steady decline from teenage years onward. In contrast, crystallized intelligence, since it is primarily dependent on learning and acculturation, is assumed to show larger increase (up to late adulthood) and, if extrapolated into old age, only a slight decline thereafter. These differential patterns became evident in former studies of *Schaie and Strother* (1968a, b) and *Nesselroade, et al.* (1972).

But looking at the 14-year follow-up studies (*Schaie et al.*, 1973; *Schaie and Labouvie-Vief,* 1974), the distinct changes in these different dimensions are no longer unequivocal. On the background of the before mentioned different age patterns for the VS and PS of the HAWIE/WAIS and with the assumption that the VS measures something at least partly like crystallized intelligence (*Savage et al.*, 1973; *Savage and Britton,* 1968) and the performance part (and the CPM administered in the BLSA without time limit) some kind of fluid intelligence, the expectations go in the following directions: for the verbal part: at most generational/cohort differences with the implication of no substantial age differences, and, if at all, slight age *changes;* for the performance part and particulary for the CPM: barely any generational/cohort differences, but clear age differences in respect to decline within the cohorts as a corollary of the decrease of biologically mediated functions. Information about these topics can be gained by application of the sequential strategies. In addition it is possible to make some inferences about test effects/testwiseness because control groups from a separate gerontological study in 1968 and genuine matched controls within the BLSA in 1972 are available.

Structural Aspects

One main problem in long-term comparisons of this kind – not merely in the cognitive area – is raised by the invariance of measurement instruments over time (*Baltes and Nesselroade,* 1970, 1973; *Bentler,* 1973; *Harwood and Naylor,* 1971; *Nesselroade et al.*, 1972; *Rudinger,* 1972a–c, 1975; *Schaie,* 1972a, b, 1973; *Schaie and Gribbin,* 1975). Scrutiny of this delicate problem within the BLSA yielded some results which are in contradiction to often cited previous findings. Our outcomes may be associated to two questions: (1) Does cross-sectional comparison between our younger (age 60–69) and older (age 70–79) group show differences with respect to intellectual pattern? (2) Are there changes within the period of 5 or 7 years in the intellectual pattern of these two groups and, if so, are there different shapes of these changes? The investigation of (quanti-)structural changes and differences (in the intellectual pattern) seems a topic of increasing interest (*Baltes and Labouvie,* 1973; *Baltes and Nesselroade,* 1970, 1973; *Botwinick,* 1970; *Buss,* 1974a–c; *Horn,* 1970; *Nesselroade,* 1970; *Reinert,* 1970).

Striving to find a common denominator for the different results of the various existing studies, it must first of all be stated that these results are attained by various intelligence tests and by different variants of factor analysis – not to speak of the diverse methods for securing the number of interpretable factors. The existing data do not seem to be invariant from a methodological viewpoint.

Nevertheless, *Botwinick* (1970), trying a synopsis, wrote that, with increasing age, intellectual organization is affected by memory deficit, according to studies carried out previously. *Thomae and Lehr* (1973) state that the results of *Balinsky's* (1941) early study can also be confirmed by recent studies, where an integration of intellectual pattern is evident with increasing age (indicated by a decreasing number of factors; see also *Reinert,* 1970; *Baltes and Labouvie,* 1973). With reference to these and other studies not mentioned here, we got the following results: after the usual routine (correlation analysis, linearity test, varimax rotation, some tests for the number of interpretable factors) and similarity rotations, we got two factors in each of the MPs for both 'age groups'.

For the time being, these two factors explained between 50 and 58% of the total variance. This two-factor solution has a general average similarity of 0.97 for all the analyses. The main variables loaded by the first factor in all the analyses are: general information, comprehension, arithmetic, and similarity. They happen to be the variables with the highest communalities in this case. This consistent framework is responsible for the similarity coefficients between groups and between times in the range 0.993–0.888. The main variables loaded by the second factor in all analyses are: digit symbol, block design, and object assembly. The similarity coefficients for the second factor are a little lower, but sufficient for accepting similarity.

To summarize, we have one factor of the HAWIE which explains 28.8–34% of the total variance and which is characterized by verbal tests ('knowledge and comprehension in treatment of verbal material'). The second factor, explaining 20–28.5% of total variance, is made up of nonverbal tests ('perceptual and spatial organization'). There is high similarity of factor patterns between our two age groups at the same MP as well as within the groups over time.

If we compare these results with the outcomes of other studies (*Riegel,* 1960; *Riegel and Riegel,* 1959; *Savage and Britton,* 1968; *Savage et al.,* 1973), the small number of factors reported here is surprising. Before we discuss the dedifferentiation or integration or, negatively, the deficit or decrease in our sample, it seems necessary to check critically the results of studies presented up to now. Individual decisions of the investigator enter into every factor analysis study. Factor analysis is an instrument which demands such decisions at several points: communalities, cut-off points for factor numbers, rotation variants, amounts of loadings, etc.

We have reanalyzed and checked some former studies using this critical approach, and we have added results from other own studies. The factor analysis techniques remained constant for about 25 analyses. We do not pretend that our decisions are absolutely right. Yet they are absolutely consistent in contrast to the practice of adopting results without noting the different methods which lead necessarily to different results.

Result of our efforts: all these studies constantly yielded only the two factors mentioned above applying uniform extraction, rotation, and interpretation criteria (*Schick et al.*, 1972; *Rudinger,* 1975). With respect to this outcome, even *Balinsky*'s (1941) early results, which have had an important influence on the following factor analysis research with the Wechsler scales and on development of the integration hypothesis with increasing age, are artifacts. In our opinion, this seems a strong support to the crucial objection that the WAIS/HAWIE, which is largely based upon *Spearman*'s notion of general factor, is 'misused' in the examination particulary of structural change characteristics (*Reinert,* 1970; *Baltes and Labouvie,* 1973).

Interindividual Differences in Change Patterns

In the following paragraphs the results of design 1 (case II ANOVA) are commonly valid for 5- and 7-year intervals as long as these two longitudinal substudies, which of course are based on different sample sizes, are not explicitly separated.

Age/Cohorts

The main effects of the factor age/cohort, averaged over 5 and 7 years, have already been mentioned in connection with the cross-sectional results. The cohorts do not differ in the VS, the interaction 'age/cohort x MP' does not reach usual significance levels and the explained proportions of variance are also not substantial (between 0 and 2.5%). That means that the performances in the verbal subtests of the two cohorts remain in the same relation to each other. This fact, however, allows no conclusion about the direction and extent of the main effect 'time'. It merely indicates that time has the same effect on the performance of both cohorts. This 'time' effect on VS reaches the 1-percent significance level. The inspection of means makes it clear that there is a one-point decline in VS from MP I (51.7) to MP III (50.8) and a two-point decline from MP I (51.5) to MP IV (49.6). This drop of about one or two points is a significant one, but, on the other hand, 'time' explains just 1% of the total variance expressed by a measure of practical significance. Similar findings, by the way, were obtained by a variance analysis 'subjects x subtests x time' for two MPs (*Rudinger,* 1971a).

The variance analyses with the PS as dependent variable show different results for the two longitudinal substudies. The ANOVA for the 5-year interval yielded significant F ratios for the main effect 'cohorts/age groups' and for the interaction 'age/cohort x time'. This significant main effect disappears in the ANOVA for the time interval of 7 years. The stable interaction refers also to different change patterns in this time span. While the younger cohort shows improving PS at least till MP IV (test effects?) and deteriorates then to MP V, the older cohort continuously declines till MP V. These partly opposite trends, of course, restrict the interpretation of the main effects 'age/cohort' and 'time', since they are based upon comparisons of means which conceal existing differences by averaging over modifying influences. As a consequence, the time effect shows no significance. The opposite trends have been graded to a curve that signals constancy of PS for the total sample.

In order to rule out the disguising test effects we have replaced the HAWIE VS and PS of the longitudinal sample by the corresponding scores of the controls tested the first time in 1972 (MP V). By this tentative approach we got plausible and unequivocal results. Performance scores are more sensitive to age changes in both cohorts, older cohorts show higher deterioration rates than the younger cohorts, especially in the performance part.

With FS as the dependent variable, the differences between cohorts and the interaction 'cohort/age x time' over 5 years do not reach conventional significance levels on account of substantial error terms 'between' and 'within'. Considering the 7-year interval, however, cohort-specific developmental patterns seem to turn up with regard even to FS. The interaction 'cohort/age group x time' gets substantial, a consequence of the greater sensibility of this variance analysis model with increasing repeated measures.

With regard to fluid intelligence as reflected by the variable CPM score, the two cohorts under study show a general decrease from the second to the fifth MP, but there is no age/cohort difference for the reduced longitudinal sample and no interaction which could be proved by statistical routine.

Replacing the dependent scores at the MP V of the longitudinal sample through the independent scores of the controls again intensifies this decline – a further hint that the testwiseness counteracts a general decline.

Social Conditions (Educational Level, SES)

There is no interaction between educational level and any other factor. The average large extent of variance this factor accounted for (about 20%) has already been reported in connection with the cross-sectional results. Since an interaction 'educational level x time' does not emerge, it is evident that each educational level retains its relative position through 5 years compared with the other groups in VS as well as in PS.

Similarly, differential developmental patterns could not be found for the different SES groups (high/low). The performances of persons in good life conditions remain clearly better than those of persons with lower SES. The proportion of variance explained by the SES factor is also quite considerable (about 15% in the PS, about 20% in the VS; see also *Grombach,* 1975).

Sex

The performance level differences between the sexes in favor of the men (especially in the verbal part!) remain stable over a time interval of 5 years. However, the (nonsignificant) tendency of the test performances of men and women to converge with passing time becomes quite clear in the once more reduced longitudinal sample from MP I to MP V: men show continuously decreasing performances in both test parts, women in general hold or even improve their level such that the men's lead in intellectual functioning is not at all as clear at MP V as at the beginning of the study.

TS and XS Analyses

HAWIE Results

We rearranged the BLSA sample in nine cohorts comprehending the mean birth years ordered from 1890 to 1906 in 2-year steps. This is the first dimension for the following analyses. The second dimension is the time of measurement. For these dependent (repeatedly measured) BLSA samples it is only possible according to the Schaie design to compute XS variance analyses and gross-longitudinal gradients and, of course, average cross-sectional gradients.

In addition to this sample, there exists an independent sample drawn in 1968 and consisting of 180 persons from another gerontological study performed by the Bonn team in Münster (*Schmitz-Scherzer et al.,* 1974), quite comparable to the Bonn sample with respect to the essential social criteria. This independent sample is arranged in 7 cohorts from 1890 to 1902 in 2-year steps. Now it is possible to apply two sequential strategies: XS and TS analyses. In this way we will also get at least some 'cross-sectional' information about testwiseness within the repeatedly measured samples.

Anticipating some results, it seems remarkable that the analyses with the factor scores estimated for the two mentioned factors as dependent variables brought the same results as the corresponding analyses with the test scores. Therefore, we will confine ourselves to a selection of findings with the test scores.

Verbal Part

The variance analyses 'cohort x time' yielded no cohort effects and no 'cohort x time' interaction, but significant negative time effects amounting to -0.94 for the two MPs (1966, 1968) and -0.48 averaged for the three MPs (1966, 1968, 1970). From the fact of no interaction 'cohort by time' in the XS analyses it is deducible that there are no significant age differences, i. e. no significant age changes. But if neither cohort nor age differences exist, then, according to the

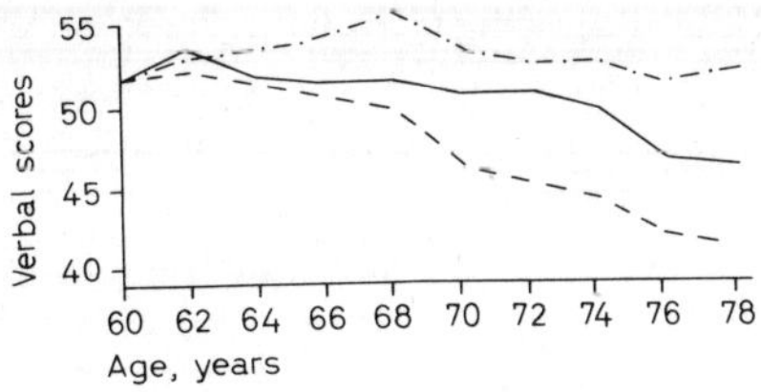

Fig. 1. Cross-sectional (–), estimated projected gross-longitudinal (– – –) and net-age change (–•–) gradients for verbal part of HAWIE constructed on the base of dependent BLSA sample.

logic of the model, it is possible to apply $Td_{k.xs}$ to estimate the time difference (needed in equation 10, *Schaie,* 1970). With this estimation of Td it is possible to construct a 'net-age change gradient' also for these dependent samples. These net-age gradients, however, are rather similar, almost identical to the averaged cross-sectional gradients (fig. 1).

The gross-longitudinal gradients, on the other hand, lie below the cross-sectional gradients, because they are loaded with the negative environmental impact. The nonsignificant cross-sectional differences reflect nothing else than the (nonsignificant) age/maturational differences in this area of cognitive functioning.

At this point we derive from these longitudinal findings that decrement in verbal scores is neither primarily age-related nor closely bound to health condition – by the way, the result of covariance-XS-analyses – but can be attributed to some unspecified negative environmental impact. It should be remembered that this conclusion does not yet pay regard to the problem of testwiseness of the BLSA sample.

The following analyses with the *independent* samples will give some explanation about this point. The XS and the TS analyses brought no cohort effects, no time effects, no age effects, no interactions at all.

The time lag estimations are quite substantial (-1.89 in XS, -1.43 in TS analyses) but, as mentioned, not significant. This relatively larger time lag than in the dependent samples leads to a steeper gross-longitudinal age gradient for the chosen cohort 1902. It is the retest effect, even though not significant as detected by a 'cross-sectional' testwiseness check, which is responsible for the differences between the gross-longitudinal gradients of dependent and independent samples, because this effect is, so to speak, a positive environmental impact. Removing all environmental impacts (positive and negative) leads to very similiar net-age gradients for both samples, which means no significant differences within the same cohort over time attributable to aging effects (fig. 2).

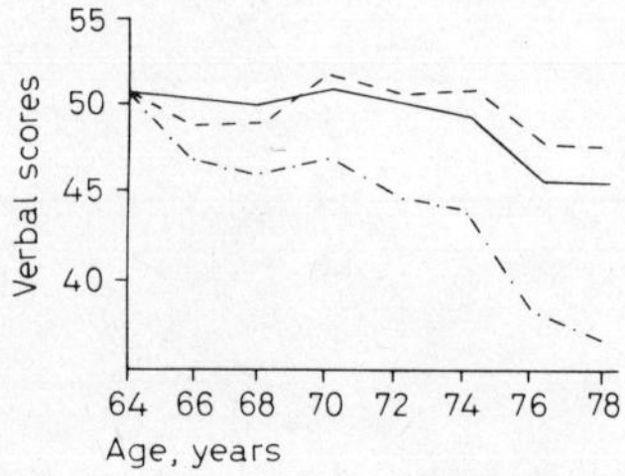

Fig. 2. Cross-sectional (–), estimated projected gross-longitudinal (–•–) and net-age change (–––) gradients for verbal part of HAWIE constructed on the base of independent samples (BLSA and Münster).

The last step according to the hypothesis stated at the beginning is the computation of cohort gradients, to illustrate the ability of all cohorts pre- and postdicted to a certain age. We chose the youngest age of the independent sample (64 years) as the basis for comparison. The cohorts under study here (from 1890 to 1902) show no net difference; all cohorts at the same age level have had or will have the same ability level measured by verbal scores of HAWIE.

Performance Part

In XS analyses we got no significant cohort effects within the dependent Bonn samples (nevertheless the factor 'cohorts' explains about 10% of total variance), no time effect and no interactions. The average time-lag estimation from XS is +0.40 (!) for the time from 1966 to 1968, and +0.30 from 1966 to 1970, an index of a positive environmental impact. As discussed with regard to verbal scores, the undifferentiated environmental impact here has at least two components: the test effect (easy to define as environmental influence, too) and the residual nondefined impacts. The ratio of these components can be indicated by the 'cross-sectional check' of test effects: testwiseness seems to play an important role, because the main effect of practice level is highly significant. More specifically, that means that persons repeatedly measured with the performance part get a bonus of about two points by their knowledge of and familiarity with the test. This is the reason for the unexpected atypical gross-longitudinal gradients with a positive slope (fig. 3). The suggestion is that a decrement proportion attributable to negative environmental influences is compensated by a greater incremental part caused by test familiarity.

No matter how atypical and biased the longitudinal gradients of the dependent samples may be, the effect of general health status in the area of cognitive functioning can nevertheless be demonstrated by covariance analyses with health as covariate: positive, i.e. ascending gradients get more ascendant, descending gradients less descendant, because with statistical control of health status a negative exacerbatory influence now is cancelled out.

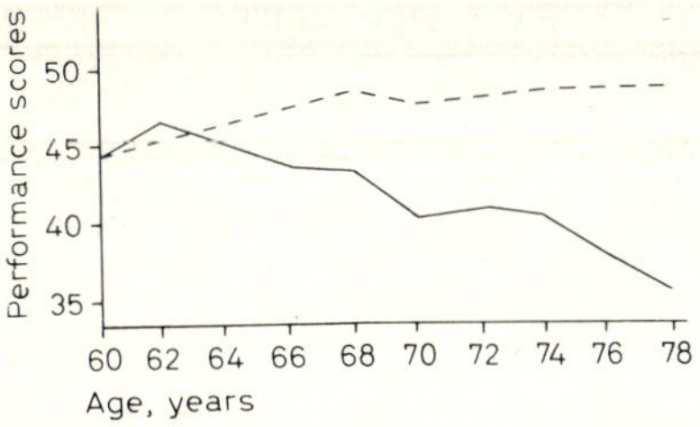

Fig. 3. Cross-sectional (–) and estimated projected gross-longitudinal (–––) gradients for performance part of HAWIE constructed on the base of dependent BLSA sample.

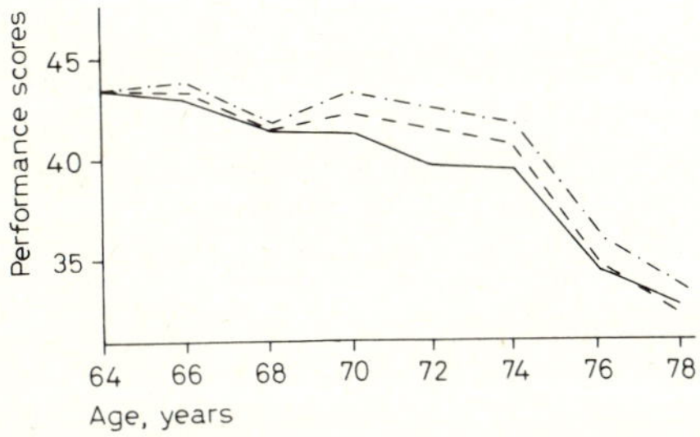

Fig. 4. Cross-sectional (–), estimated projected gross-longitudinal (–•–) and net-age change (–––) gradients for performance part of HAWIE constructed on the base of independent samples (BLSA and Münster).

The next task is to control the testwiseness bias by the independent samples. The TS analyses brought a significant age effect and no time effect (only –0.22). For computing the longitudinal gradient and revealing other possible sources of variance it was necessary to perform the XS analyses. The variance analyses yielded a significant effect on the factor 'cohorts', but no significant time effect, although the time difference is about –1.73; in both analyses, no interaction 'cohort or age by time' was found. Age and cohort seem to be the two relatively independent sources of variance. This result has to become evident also from the gradients. The gross-longitudinal gradient (including the small negative environmental impact) is quite identical with the cross-sectional gradient (fig. 4). Even after removing the small negative impact of environment, the net-age gradient does not differ significantly from the cross-sectional gradient, i.e. the cross-sectional differences for these variables are a function of maturational (age) changes alone.

This coincidence of the two gradients serves as a rule as proof of no cohort differences, because *if* there are environmental and/or generation differences, then discrepancies between the two gradients would be expected. But why, if the TS shows no cohort differences, does the XS, on the other hand, show substantial cohort differences? It is an opportune argument to say that these cohort differences are not reliable because, as TS shows, the assumptions for XS are not met. This conclusion is supported by 'estimating the cohort gradient at age 64 for all cohorts under study.

CPM Results

The Raven test was administered at MPs II, IV and V as an index for fluid intelligence. These test results shall now be discussed. Between MP II and V there was an interval of 5 years (1967–1972), to which the following findings refer. The longitudinal sample for this 5-year period included 110 persons. The drop-out process will be commented on later.

Sample Composition

In order to control the well-known effects within studies with repeated measurement, we drew a comparable independent sample in 1972 (MP V) of about 60 persons, who were tested with the same procedures. In this manner we obtained performance changes which are not seriously confounded by sample attrition and practice influences. The social characteristics of the longitudinal sample have not changed essentially since the study was started (*Schmitz-Scherzer,* 1975c). By the way, this group of retestees – constituting the longitudinal sample – was separately compared to dropouts with psychological reasons and to the nonsuvivors, who can be said to have dropped out for biological reasons (chap. xxx). For our purposes, however, it will be more important to find out if the longitudinal sample, reduced by several attrition processes, is a selected sample in respect to the dependent variable (i. e. the Raven scores).

It could be shown that the two before mentioned cohorts are indeed biased subsamples: persons tested between 1967 and 1972 (i.e. those who remained in the study for 5 years) had already achieved better CPM results in 1967 than those who dropped out later, after 1967 or 1968/69.

Our present study covers a smaller age range, a subset of the range included in *Schaie*'s study. Compared to *Horn*'s cross-sectional study, we begin with an age (60 years) where the study of *Horn* ends.

Design and Data Analyses

CPM data are available from the BLSA sample tested twice (1967 and 1972) and an independent cross-sectional sample drawn in 1972. Therefore, we could combine TS and XS analyses according to the Schaie 'General Developmental Model' i.e. 'age x time of measurement' and ,cohort x time of measurement'. Prior to performing the analyses of variance, samples were arranged into 5-year intervals ranging from 1905 to 1890, the mean birth years.

Results

The XS analyses of variance, not presented here, showed time effects ($Td_{k.xs}$ indep = –4.03, dep = –1.7) but no cohort effects. In the XS design this

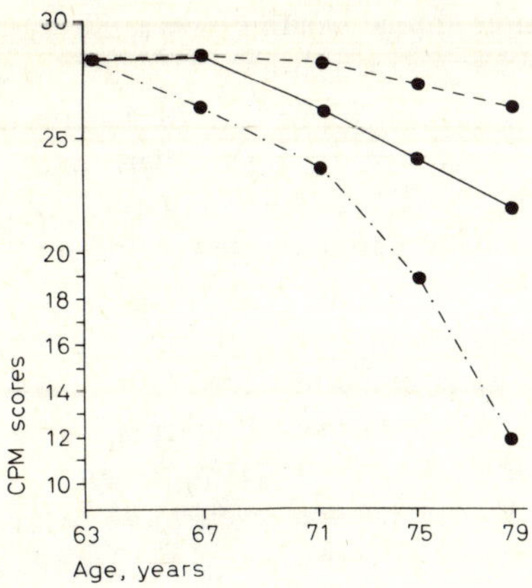

Fig. 5. Cross-sectional (– – –) and estimated projected gross-longitudinal gradients for CPM scores, constructed on the base of dependent BLSA sample (–) and independent samples (BLSA and control group; ·–·).

time of measurement effect represents a genuine longitudinal change, which is obviously extenuated by positive environmental impact, that is, testwiseness in the dependent sample. In general, the gradients show – especially for the dependent samples – the typical relations between subsequent cross-sectional measures and within-cohort gradients for this intellectual dimension. The independent samples show specific within-cohort age effects, i.e. the age changes increase for the elder cohorts. This trend has become evident in our own results obtained by the HAWIE performance part and psychomotor tests, as well as in the findings of *Schaie* and his associates. This statment becomes even more distinct in the light of the following consideration. The comparison of the estimated cross-sectional gradients with the estimated longitudinal gradients in figure 5 demonstrates the well-known shape of projected 'development' in the area of fluid intelligence.

Concluding Remarks

Evaluating the most recent results of several important longitudinal studies – Human Development Studies, Berkeley and Oakland; New England Study; her own Twin Study; Duke Study; Iowa State Study; Guidance Study – *Jarvik* (1973, p. 65) summarizes:
'Despite differences in the composition of the samples with regard to age, intelligence, education, socio-economic background, and other relevant variables,

there appears to be at least one common thread leading toward a cohesive pattern of intellectual functioning in the later years of life. – That thread seems to be a remarkable stability of verbal scores – whenever health has been preserved – accompanied by a relentlessly progressive decline in performance on speeded tasks. Thus our longitudinal studies have led us to rediscover the classical pattern of aging! And this pattern is evident under a wide variety of circumstances.'

This statement is also qualified for characterizing our own longitudinal findings. The trend, roughly indicated already by several cross-sectional studies (*Botwinick,* 1967; *Green,* 1969; *Riegel and Riegel,* 1972), that with increasing age – as a process being represented by time elapsed in our ANOVA design 1 – the differences in performance between age groups become even more distinct is caused by different change-patterns in the performance part (described as ANOVA interaction 'cohort/age by time'). That it makes sense, despite the justifiably reserved attitude of some authors (*Baltes and Labouvie,* 1973; *Schaie and Gribbin,* 1975), to separate between verbal and performance part, by the way, stable factorial dimension over occasions, cohorts and ages (*Rudinger,* 1975), could be illustrated by the application of XS and TS analyses in the BLSA in order to describe differential patterns of development also in old age.

In the field represented by the verbal part of HAWIE – some kind of crystallized intelligence (?), see *Savage and Britton* (1968) – we got no substantial age changes, but also no cohort differences. It seems a partly atypical result for this area of cognitive functioning, but remembering the relatively limited cohort range in the BLSA in comparison to other studies, these findings seem to more or less conform to theoretical expectation. The main result for the performance part: age maturational bounded decrement even for this age level of BLSA, scarcely environmental impact, and no substantial generational differences seems to fit into the theory of visuo-motor flexibility (*Nesselroade et al.,* 1972) and/or fluid intelligence. The analysis with Raven's CPM, a measure of fluid intelligence (*Cunningham et al.,* 1975), yielded more unequivocal results without any uneasiness with theoretical status of intelligence measures as HAWIE, especially having ruled out the speed component by applying this test without any time limit. The results clearly show age-dependent changes in the field of fluid intelligence. This casts no doubt on the validity of *Schaie*'s conclusion emphasizing that this presumably biologically based slowing might at least in part be linked to specific cultural-historical contingencies. For one thing, our generalizations are based on an age range from 60 years on and for another we also got cohort-specific age changes. They may be less dramatic and less puzzling than *Schaie*'s second follow-up results, for they show the same direction, but they do exist. In other words, the fact that in the BLSA changes in fluid intelligence are best described by the age component does not have full explanatory power.

But age and generation are not the only factors that can be used in order to discover interindividual change patterns. The BLSA itself includes a lot of other possible modifiers of aging functions, of which we have selected only a small sample: health, sex, sociocultural background, occupation, educational level, global index of socioeconomic status. General health turned out to be an essential source of performance decrease in old age. Because of increasing probability of illness at higher age, it is clear that different performance levels within the age groups also have to be explained by different health conditions. *Correll and Rokosz* (1966), for example, conclude that performance tests are especially sensitive to differences in general health (*Wilkie and Eisdorfer,* 1973). However, the relatively minor role of the health factor in our study may be attributed to the following facts: our rating index for general health status is a relatively undifferentiated global measure. The validity of this argument has been illustrated in a study of *Angleitner et al.* (1973), where the superiority of a set of some detailed medical measures over a global health index could be demonstrated by multiple regression techniques. On the other hand, the Bonn sample seems to be very homogeneous with respect to health status. But that does not preclude interpretation of our results with *Birren*'s (1964) categories; he distinguishes between 'age-related' changes (including the primary process of aging, as also became evident in our study in the speed-tests of the performance part) and 'health-related' changes. The latter affect all cognitive functions and, therefore, affect the verbal intelligence tasks in the same manner. The analysis of the effect of concomitant *changes* in health condition on *changes* in intellectual performance, however, ought yet to be done – at least for the BLSA.

A very high degree of interindividual variability of intellectual performance is due to the sociocultural background. This has been demonstrated in several studies (for summary, see *Granick and Friedmann,* 1973) as well as in the BLSA! But are the different levels necessarily associated with differential change patterns over time? Within the BLSA, the answer for the time intervals of 5 and 7 years is no. The clear differences in favor of groups with higher SES – indicated by educational level, occupational status, or by a general SES index – remain constant at least over 5 and 7 years, i. e. there is no differential development in diverse groups with different intellectual levels conditioned by quite different life histories and biographical influences (*Schoenfeldt,* 1973), with different stimulating environments throughout life (*Loewe,* 1970; *Birren and Woodruff,* 1973). In this connection, it seems worth mentioning that in the BLSA sample the knowledge of the socioeconomic status of the *parents* of our old-age sample allows a prediction of intellectual status of the aged people about 12.8% better than chance. Findings of this kind call attention to the need for molar ecological approaches in a life-span perspective in order to explain 'extent and kind of change taking place in a particular characteristic' (*Bloom,* 1964, p. 209). In this connection, it has to be emphazised that the fruitful concepts of enrichment and deprivation ought not to be confined to studies of institutionalization effects. (*Weinstock and Bennett,* 1969). Within this widened frame of reference the interrelationship of 'intelligence-education-occupation' plays a very important and probably crucial role for our results in the sense of a self-reinforcing system during development from youth to old age. Education, occupation and sex explains the variance in HAWIE performances to a greater degree than age (*Britton et al.,* 1967). Even in a sample (n=670) in the age range 20–90 years, as much variance could be explained by educational level as by 'age' (*Rudinger,* 1974).

Many studies and theories deal with the relevance of test performance dependence on education just for different age groups, or, more precisely, generations (*Anastasi,* 1967; *Birren and Morrison,* 1961; *Granick and Friedman,* 1967; *Kuhlen,* 1963). Result: on the one hand, a retreat from a biologically oriented intelligence model (with changes of performance in analogy to organic changes) in favor of a sociocultural intelligence concept; on the other hand, statement of critical gaps in assessing intelligence in old age. These gaps make it clear that the problem of finding criteria for describing intelligence in old age is not yet solved either (*Bijou,* 1971; *Birren,* 1964; *Fischer,* 1973; *Humphrey,* 1971; *Tulkin and Konner,* 1973).

Interpreting the performance differences between the sexes in favor of male subjects, it must be kept in mind that there is a distinguishing feature in our sample that presents a social difference between the two sex groups: the formerly or presently practiced occupation with its often emphasized opportunities of stimulation and training; 49% of the women in our longitudinal sample have never learned any occupation. Only 11% practiced their occupation at the time of our first investigation. Needless to say, all men were professionally trained, and 36% are still employed. The differences in the tests, which become most clear in the verbal part, may be explained by the daily demands being congruent with the 'verbal' skills of the tests, a problem, which we believe touches again the discussion on the validity of assessing intelligence in adulthood and old age. The differential changes over time (at least for the time interval of 7 years) raise some problems in evaluating them. One possible explanation might be that a stronger positive selection process has taken place within the female group, an interaction 'sex x dropout process', another that women needed a longer time to overcome their deficit in familiarity with achievement situations as test sessions usually are, that they succeeded an emotional adaptation (*Thomae,* 1969), an interaction 'sex x adaptation to test situation'.

Furthermore, attention has to be called to the possibility that differential 'aging' patterns associated with initial ability level (tied to sex and especially to the sociocultural variables) may be polluted by regression effects (*Baltes et al,* 1972; *Baltes and Labouvie,* 1973; *Eisdorfer,* 1963; *Rudinger,* 1971a). Admittedly this rival hypothesis has yet to be scrutinized. Besides this last mentioned rival explanation there are in general some additional interpretations and undesired components of change, as pointed out repeatedly by *Baltes and Labouvie* (1973): sample and population composition, terminal change, age-and cohort-specific validities of measurement instruments.

To begin with the last one: cross-occasion and cross-cohort factor analyses suggest factor pattern invariance of HAWIE, a support for unchanged validity. The first and the second problem will be handled in chapter x. For the moment, just a brief note. As demonstrated for the longitudinal sample (n=110) measured three times with Raven's CPM, this sample is indeed a positively biased one with regard to the dependent variable. This positively biased sample might simulate changes in a psychological variable as already shown by *Baltes and Labouvie* (1973). Another problem, to which *Baltes et al.* (1971) drew attention, is the possibility of interaction 'cohort by selection', which can be ruled out only by means of longitudinal sequences. In our study we found such cohort differences in dropout effects on the dependent variable CPM score.

Similar effects could be traced with regard to the dependent variables VS, PS, FS (see also chapter x; *Rudinger and Schmitz-Scherzer,* 1976). Probably it is this attrition effect which makes some differences (main effects, e.g., age/cohort on PS for four MPs) disappear or which levels other differences (e.g. sex on intellectual performance). In general, this means that the present results of the longitudinal study are based on a selected 'elite' sample.

But this need not mean that the results are generally useless, as *Schaie et al.*, (1973) and *Schaie and Labouvie-Vief* (1974) have shown by using dependent and independent samples in their second follow-up studies to the original 1956 study. Comparing the outcomes of these two studies, they concluded: 'although we know the longitudinal samples . . . (are) . . . positively selected in comparison to the independent controls, the pattern of change nevertheless appeared to be generalizable to a wider proportion of the general population' (*Schaie et al.*, 1973, p. 164) – a generalization which may be admissible to some degree also for the BLSA sample.

Contr. hum. Dev., vol. 3, pp. 36–50 (Karger, Basel 1976)

IV. Psychomotor Performance and Reaction Speed in Old Age

Franz Josef Mathey

Introduction

In order to get a record of psychomotor or sensorimotor performance using an instrument particularly sensitive to influence caused by age, a choice reaction time experiment was carried out at all measurement sessions of the Bonn Longitudinal Study of Aging (BLSA). The strong influence of age on choice reaction time measures of psychomotor performance is well known from relevant publications on the subject (*Heegner,* 1957; *Welford and Birren,* 1965). The special experimental task used in our study also intended to provide information on the susceptibility of aging subjects to stress in a psychomotor achievement task. To this end we incorporated numerous and highly variable perceptual and reaction variants under standardized conditions in our experimental design.

Experimental results from a 7-year observation period of the BLSA are presently available. During this period, each subject was tested at five measurement points, namely the first testing session and two annual follow-up measurements (1965, 1966, 1967), one follow-up study after a 2-year interval (1969), and a final follow-up study after a 3-year interval (1972). At the last measurement point, additional data were gathered from a sample of newcomers or so-called investigation twins consisting of persons with the same age distribution as in the longitudinal sample.

Preliminary data evaluation from the first years of the study had already shown that the results of the relative complex multiple choice reaction task not only reflect age and sex influences to a high degree, but are also very closely connected to other psychological, physical, and social characteristics of the subjects. In other words, the results of the experiment with the choice reaction time task depend in part on personal conditions such as complex achievement dispositions and other determinants of achievement among the tested persons. In order to clarify these connections as well as the observed age and sex differences, a measure of the simple, so-called 'absolute' reaction time to simple visual and acoustic stimuli was included in the last two measurement sessions (1969, 1972). Thus, a longitudinal comparison of reaction time data from before and after a 2-year interval was made possible.

The measurement of simple reaction time was intended to provide data as free as possible from complications due to stimuli presentation, stimuli perception, and stimuli reaction, which are unavoidable and intentional influences in choice reaction time tasks. In addition, simple reaction time serves as a measure of psychomotor performance in its most elementary form. Using these data, further comparisons in regard to age and sex differences and other aspects such as psychological, physical, or social variables could be carried out.

This procedure holds promise of providing new information on possible parallels between psychomotor performance on choice reaction time measures and on simple reaction time measures. Current publications on this subject indicate that such correlations cannot be taken for granted (*Heegner,* 1957). Above all, differences are pointed out in the internal psychological activation systems engaged in processing the stimuli. Psychomotor or sensorimotor multiple choice reactions can be regarded as 'reflected reactions' of a rather nature (*Heegner,* 1957). They occur under conditions where the character of the stimuli or the nature of the reactions makes the operation of conscious or nearly conscious processes necessary. Complex reaction time tests usually consist of responding in particular ways to various sensory constellations presented as stimuli. The response pattern often calls for a combination of different reactions such as hand and foot pressure on different keys. Measures of simple reaction time, on the other hand, generally require only a minimum of conscious activity. *Heegner* (1957) describes them as 'reflectoric reactions', and they are closely related to the physiological reflex. Measures of simple reaction time can therefore be treated as indicators of underlying neurological reflex functioning and possibly reflect the influence of other physical conditions.

Psychomotor Performance as Choice Reaction Time

Procedure

In this study we used the Kieler determination instrument developed by *Mierke.* The task of the subject is to respond to flashing colored light signals by pushing buttons of corresponding color. For two additional light signals the correct responses consist of pushing designated foot pedals. The speed of the signal sequence can be varied, allowing for steady acceleration up to and beyond the point where a decline in performance is registered.

Stress was introduced in a manner contrived to satisfy conditions of both standardization and adaptability to individual differences. First, subjects accustomed themselves to working the apparatus at low-speed signal sequence. Then the signal sequence speed gradually increased until the level at which the subject responded correctly to 50% of the stimuli could be determined.

Empirical results reported by *Hoyos* (1960a, b) and *Kottenhoff* (1959) indicate that even a slight acceleration above the so-called 50-percent reaction level usually leads to clear signs of stress. In our study, considerable stress was induced by exceeding the individual 50-percent reaction level first by one speed level and then by two. Following the first trial, the test was repeated twice without interruption. The standardized stress testing took place three times in all.

Quantitative Results

The following results are based on the observed 50-percent reaction levels given in seconds. These units refer to the time during which a constant number of stimuli were presentated (circulation period). Prolonged circulation periods, therefore, mean worse performance, and shorter circulation periods mean better performance.

Means and Standard Deviations

Table I gives the mean performance results for different samples in the study. Table II shows the standard deviations. Tables I and II also contain corresponding data from a sample of university students between 20 and 30 years of age. Figure 1 is a graphic illustration of the material presented in table I. This presentation facilitates identification of longitudinal developments in performance over the retesting sessions. It also shows differences between the various samples more clearly.

Age-Related Performance Differences

The clearest performance differences are those occurring between the various age groups. As can be seen from table I and figure 1, these differences are equally great at all five measurement points. At all measurement points they achieve significance at better than the 1-percent niveau. The most striking performance difference is found for the investigation twins, tested in 1972 for the first time. This is most likely due to the lack of previous experience with the choice reaction time testing procedure among the twins as compared to the longitudinal sample.

Particularly interesting differences were discovered between the standard deviations of performance scores, shown in table II. These differences, equally observable at all five measurement points, are even more distinct than those between the means in table I. This result shows a much stronger dissociation of scores in the sample of the 70- to 80-year olds, which means that individual differences in psychomotor performance are much more widespread for this

Table I. Longitudinal development of the mean circulation periods, in which 50% correct reactions were gained in the choice reaction time task (Mierke apparatus)[1]

	Measurement point					Twins (1972)
	I (1965)	II (1966)	III (1967)	IV (1969)	V (1972)	
Men[2]						
Aged 60–70	178 (47)	184 (44)	175 (39)	183 (37)	213 (34)	230 (13)
Aged 70–80	214 (50)	209 (49)	203 (44)	212 (40)	241 (24)	286 (11)
Women[2]						
Aged 60–70	192 (50)	195 (42)	187 (47)	192 (37)	225 (32)	225 (21)
Aged 70–80	233 (42)	228 (38)	232 (33)	226 (26)	267 (27)	287 (9)

1 Values for university students aged 20–30 (1967): men, 147 (n=50); women, 155 (n=50).
2 Number of subjects tested is given in parentheses.

Table II. Longitudinal development of the standard deviations for the performances in the choice reaction time task (Mierke apparatus)[1]

	Measurement point					Twins (1972)
	I (1965)	II (1966)	III (1967)	IV (1969)	V (1972)	
Men[2]						
Aged 60–70	17.5(47)	27.2(44)	23.9(39)	35.4(37)	50.8(34)	49.5(13)
Aged 70–80	42.2(50)	30.5(49)	32.4(44)	45.5(40)	39.4(24)	65.2(11)
Women[2]						
Aged 60–70	28.5(50)	33.2(42)	27.2(47)	34.2(37)	58.5(32)	36.0(21)
Aged 70–80	40.0(42)	35.7(38)	48.0(33)	43.7(26)	52.5(27)	58.8(9)

1 Values for university students aged 20–30 (1967): men, 11.1 (n = 50); women, 12.0 (n = 50).
2 Number of subjects tested is given in parentheses.

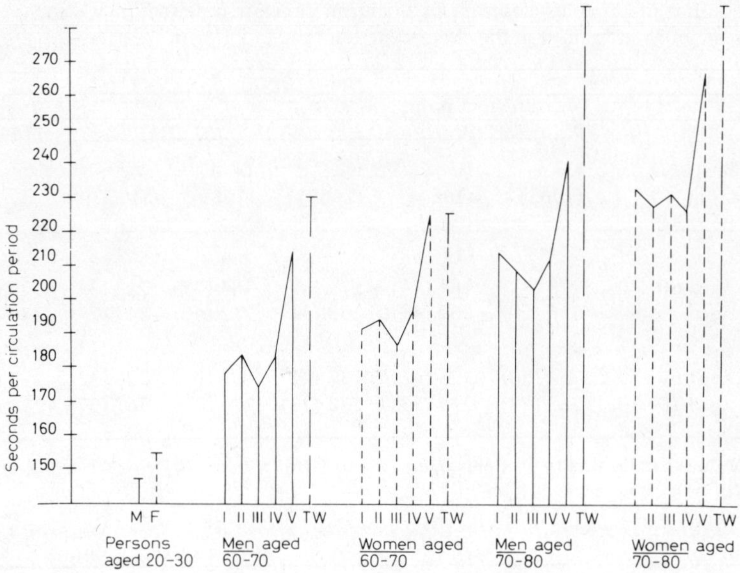

Fig. 1. Longitudinal development of the mean circulation periods, in which 50% correct reactions were gained in the choice reaction time task (Mierke apparatus). Roman numerals indicate measurement points. M = male; F = female; TW = investigation twins.

sample than among the roughly 10-year-younger sample of 60- to 70-year olds. Comparing the discrepancy between the standard deviations for the student sample (table II) and for 60- to 70-year olds with the observed difference between the two elderly samples, we find a much more marked difference between the samples of 60- to 70-year olds and 70- to 80-year olds than between 60- to 70-year olds and 20- to 30-year olds.

Sex-Related Performance Differences

Sex-related differences do not compete with the age-related performance differences, but they are discernible (tables I, II; fig. 1). At all measurement points, consistently better psychomotor performance was registered for the male subjects. Sex-related differences of this kind were particularly noticeable in the older sample of 70- to 80-year-old subjects. By far the greatest sex-related difference was found among the investigation twins, who had no training prior to their initial testing in 1972.

It should be noted, however, that sex-related differences such as those reported above are not restricted to elderly subjects. The performance differences between performance of men and women in our far younger control sample are also significant, although they are not as great as in the older age groups.

Sex-related differences in standard deviations were not very clear. The female groups tended to have somewhat higher standard deviations, but this trend cannot be observed in all samples at all measurement points.

Characteristics of Longitudinal Performance Change during the 7-Year Period of Observation

From the longitudinal development of performance, shown graphically in figure 1, it can be seen that in the first years of the study a moderate tendency towards improving performance occurred. This trend can be observed for the different age and sex groups till about the third testing, that is, during the annual retesting phase. These differences between the yearly follow-up studies are not statistically significant, however. On the contrary, computed intercorrelations point to rather high stability of performance over this 3-year period, on the whole. Age-related performance changes, which might have been expected, are apparently compensated for or surpassed to a great degree by accumulating training effects.

At the fourth measurement point in 1969, following a 2-year testing break, all age and sex groups tended to perform less well, with the exception of the 70- to 80-year-old women. For the individual groups, however, this trend was not significant.

A considerable and highly significant decrement was observed at the fifth measurement point in 1972, after a further testing interval of 3 years. This development also holds for all age and sex groups of the longitudinal sample. This decrease in the level of psychomotor performance obviously results from a combination of influences of age, here maximized by the longest testing interval of the study, and lack of practice in the intervening period. It would appear, however, that the longitudinal sample still retained some benefits of training, since the untrained twins scored significantly lower in nearly all age and sex groups (except the 60- to 70-year-old women).

Longitudinal developments as reflected by the standard deviations follow essentially the same trend described above for the means. This is especially true for development between the fourth and fifth measurement points. Here again the variation between individual performance scores increases with advancing age during the period of longitudinal observation.

The same longitudinal development described above is also to be found in a longitudinal comparison of means and standard deviations for only those subjects who were tested at every measurement point, i.e. who were on no occasion prevented by illness, death, or other reasons from participating in testing. This longitudinal core sample consisted of 100 persons in all (30 men and 28 women between 60 and 70 years of age, 23 men and 19 women above 70).

Results on the Connection between Choice Reaction Time and other Variables

Relations between Psychomotor Choice Reaction Time and Simple Reaction Time

These relations, measured at the last two measurement points, will be discussed later (cf. p. xxx). At this point we can merely note that such interrelationships are easiest to observe on the basis of reaction time following visually presented stimuli.

Table III. Correlations between choice reaction performance (Mierke apparatus) and the subtest results of the Hamburg-Wechsler Intelligence Test for Adults (HAWIE) at the 3rd measurement point of the study

		HAWIE-verbal subtests					HAWIE-perform. subtests				
		AW	AV	ZN	RD	GF	ZS	BO	BE	MT	FL
Men	60-70 y.old	–	–	–	++	–	+	–	–	–	–
	70-80 y.old	–	–	+	–	++	++	+	++	++	++
Women	60-70 y.old	++	–	–	+	++	++	++	++	++	++
	70-80 y.old	–	++	–	–	–	++	++	–	–	–

++ = highly significant (1% level)
\+ = significant (5% level)
– = not significant

AW = Allgemeines Wissen (general information)
AV = Allgemeines Verständnis (general comprehension)
ZN = Zahlen Nachsprechen (digit span)
RD = Rechnerisches Denken (arithmetic)
GF = Gemeinsamkeiten Finden (similarities)

ZS = Zahlen-Symbol-Test (coding)
BO = Bilder ordnen (picture arrangement)
BE = Bilder Ergänzen (picture completion)
MT = Mosaik-Test (block design)
FL = Figuren Legen (object assembly)

Relation between Choice Reaction Time and Intelligence

The best documented relation between psychomotor reaction time and an outside variable in our study was that between choice reaction time and intelligence. Based on scores of the Hamburg-Wechsler intelligence scale for adults (HAWIE) administered at measurement points I, III, IV and V and on the Raven colored progressive matrices test given at measurement point II, significant correlations between choice reaction time and intelligence scores were found at all measurement points. The observed variations occurring in particular age and sex groups turned out not to be homogeneous for all measurement points. Closer examination of the HAWIE results showed that this correlation not only stands up for the less language-dependent subtests, the so-called performance scale, but also for the verbal scale. Precisely this type of relationship can be interpreted as an indication that choice reaction time is a relatively complex measure related not only to narrowly defined intellectual functions but also to general intellectual capacities and flexibility, including verbal intelligence.

Similar relations can also be observed in the performance of longitudinal extreme groups although they do not (as might be expected) reach a proportionately higher degree. In this study, longitudinal extreme groups were compared by correlating intelligence scores for those subjects who consistently achieved above average or below average records on the choice reaction time task.

The high correlation between intelligence and psychomotor choice reaction time found for all measurement points in this study is not surprising. In earlier factor-analytic studies, including results obtained on the Kieler determination instrument, *Kottenhoff* (1959) found that 25% of the total variance loaded on the intelligence factor in addition to a high proportion of age variance.

Some more detailed information on the question as to which specific intellectual functions have particularly high correlations with choice reaction performance is presently available in the form of correlations for HAWIE subtest data from the third point of measurement (table III).

Correlations between Choice Reaction Time and Rating Scores on a Number of Personality Dimensions

Results from these correlations are also available. The personality ratings were undertaken for each subject immediately after individual testing at all measurement points. χ^2-Comparisons were carried out with personality ratings in the area of 'degree of activity', 'adjustment' (defined as the regulation of behavior according to the situation at hand), and 'self-control' (defined as behavior controlled in conformity to long-range goals) (*Thomae,* 1971a, b; *Simons, et al.,* 1968).

Correlation results for measurement points I, II, IV, and V are available at present. At all these measurement points, results from the total sample yielded evidence of significant correlations between choice reaction time and degree of activity in the sense that persons with above average choice reaction performance obtained higher activity ratings and those with below average choice reaction performance were rated lower on activity. This result was confirmed by a correlative comparison between longitudinal extreme groups scoring either consistently above or below average on choice reaction tasks at all five points of measurement. For ratings on the personality dimension 'self-control', a similar positive correlation was found at the first and second measurement point. For ratings of 'adjustment', a positive correlation was found solely at the first point of measurement. Findings for the age and sex groups seem to indicate that activity and self-control are related to choice reaction time among the older group of persons from 70 to 80 years of age.

Correlative Relationship between Choice Reaction Achievement and Selected Physical and Health Variables

Available data material also made it possible to investigate this relationship. Selected physical and health variables had been included in the medical part of the study. Ratings of general physical status were compared for the first two measurement points (1965 and 1966) and for the last two (1969 and 1972). In all these comparisons we found a significant relation (chi-square) for the total sample between above average performance in choice reaction tasks and very good or good general physical status. On the other hand, below average choice reaction performance and ratings of average general physical status correlated significantly. The described relation increased in a comparison of longitudinal extreme groups, which had constantly performed either above average or below average in all choice reaction tests at all five measurement points of the study.

In the first year of the study (1965) a significant correlation was found between low blood pressure and lower performance in the choice reaction task. This relation was not confirmed, however, by the results of a further correlation carried out with the data of the fifth measurement point.

Up to the present, correlational comparisons between the following physical and health variables and choice reaction performance have only been carried out for the 5th measurement point. First these variables were correlated to choice reaction performance at the same (fifth) measurement point (cross-sectional comparison). Then, further comparisons were carried out to investigate the the relations of these variables to choice reaction performance of longitudinal extreme groups consisting of such persons who had shown either above average or below average choice reaction performance at all five measurement points. Here a significant correlation was found (for the fifth year of the study) in relation to the variable 'worries about health'. Above average choice reaction performance was associated with lower preoccupation with physical troubles and vice versa. A similar correlation was found for the variables 'hearing ability' and ratings of 'subjective feeling of physical well-being'. An indicated but not yet significant correlation was found for the variables 'cardiovascular insufficiency' and 'arteriosclerosis' (low values connected with a tendency to better choice reaction performance). No correlation could be found in relation to the variables 'eyesight' and 'degree of physical motility'.

Relationship between Choice Reaction Achievement and
Selected Variables of the Social Background

This relationship has been examined for the first 2 years of the study. Significant positive correlations between choice reaction performance and the variables 'formal education', 'socioeconomic status', and 'income' occurred in the first 2 years of the study despite certain shifts in accentuation among the different age and sex groups. For the first year of the study (1965) a further significant positive correlation was found in relation to 'general satisfaction with the life situation'. A surprising but significant correlation could be observed in the first 2 years of the study with regard to some specific vocation-related activities. For the male sample it was found that the persons, who had been employed as office workers before retirement, obtained better choice reaction activities. For the male sample it was found that the persons who had been employed as office workers before retirement obtained better choice reaction on the choice reaction task than women who had not been engaged in vocational work. It can also be shown that the first group were more resistant to induced psychophysical stress.

Summary and Interpretation of the Quantitative Results

At first glance the influence of age on performance on the relatively demanding psychomotor task with limited time seems most impressive. The effect of age is much more striking than that of sex. To be sure, the sex-related performance differences were also clear, but they were also observed to a less degree in a sample composed of young adults.

A closer differentiation of the observed performance conditions shows that the influence of age and sex may not be seen as exclusive determinants. The more complex and not at all specific function of the choice reaction time seems also to have very extensive and close connections to a number of psychological, physical, and social variables. Consequently, choice reaction performance would seem to be an important indicator of smooth and intact functioning as well as general flexibility in these areas. As our results have shown, such functional relations are also relatively complex, and their influence is by no means restricted to purely neurophysiological functioning. Instead, we seem to be dealing here with physical variables of a general and practical nature, variables like the general physical status, absence of worries about health, and subjective feeling of physical well-being. These variables, in turn, are closely connected to further influence variables originating in the field of past and present social conditions like vocation, social status, and formal education. In relation to the psychological area of this study, we find above all a close connection of sensorimotor capacity to intelligence and activity of personality.

The results of psychomotr choice reaction measurements seem to reflect above all a general tendency towards flexibility and general drive and a component of general physical strength. As our quantitative results have shown directly or indirectly, such influence variables seem, independently of age, to play an important role with reference to the kind and speed of changes in important performance capacities in old age. Furthermore, our results point out the importance and relative durability of training influences related to such performance functions.

Results of Casuistic Case Studies

With the object of further supplementing our quantitative results, case histories were drawn up from the investigation materials available for members of longitudinal extreme groups, consisting of persons who had shown either above average or below average performance in all years of the study. Furthermore, the case material of those few persons who had changed from extremely good performance to bad performance in the course of the study was also evaluated casuistically. A lot of further possibilities of differentiation result from the casuistic study carried out mainly by *Monthofer* 1970. So it is indicated that being exposed to stressful influences during life, for instance, could have a positive effect on psychophysiological performance potential, if these exposures lead to enforced improvement efforts, especially of an intellectual kind. Unfavorable influences resulted, however, from prolonged exposure to extreme stress. Conditions seem to be most favorable when the problem-solving efforts take place in a subjective environment, which is relatively free from disturbances, combined with positive expectations for the future.

Positive effects were also found for persons who set themselves high standards and at the same time were content with their general life situation. Vocational change proved to be favorable if it took place voluntarily and if the person concerned was equally or more satisfied with his new vocational position. Under certain conditions, maintenance of the initial performance level by women was found to go hand in hand with high social involvement, a wide range of interests, and a wide range of social contacts. In this context, a wide range of social contacts is understood as extending beyond the circle of close friends and relatives into areas such as regular concert or theater attendance, keeping up with politics, or travelling. Contact with others proved to be most beneficial when it went smoothly and was experienced positively, for example, when contact led to the feeling of being needed. There were signs that persons who remained integrated in social groups and did not reduce their level of activity (although they may have changed it somewhat) later did quite well on tests of psychophysical capacity. Concerning the influence of physical health, it can generally be said that poor health condition had an unfavorable effect on psychomotor capacity. However, a special role must be ascribed here to subjective experience. According to the results of the casustic studies, a person's subjective assessment of his own health may in many cases be more relevant than a number of objectively stated medical diagnoses. In fact, there were cases where psychomotor performance and subjective health estimates underwent parallel declines even though the fears of deteriorating health were unfounded.

The above results sum up the major findings of casuistic studies carried out with persons whose psychomotor performance capacities were longitudinally extreme values. The results of these case studies show that casuistic investigations are often able to complement and supplement the analysis and interpretation of quantitative results by providing subtle individual insights.

Measurements of Simple Reaction Time

As described in more detail in the first paragraph (p. 37) above, the measurement of simple reaction speed was included in the fourth and fifth measurement points (1969 and 1972) in order to obtain a basic reaction measure in addition to the complex psychomotor measure of choice reaction time. Intervening variables, expecially those caused by complex psychological processes, were to be excluded as far as possible. The measurement of simple (so-called absolute) reaction speed of responses to simple acoustic and visual stimuli was taken to be an appropriate measure.

Data were gathered using *Beck*'s reaction measurement and registration apparatus, with which different experimental trials can be run to obtain measurements and continuous registration of reaction times to simple acoustic and simple visual stimuli separately. The results of the reaction time measurements carried out at the fourth and fifth measurement points of the BLSA (1969 and 1972) were available for analysis.

The results for basic reaction speed on a simple reaction task are generally similar to the results for choice reaction performance. That is, we find a definite, among the older subjects even a rising prolongation of reaction time, together with increasing standard deviation. Sex-related differences of performance were found in all age groups under study such that more prolonged reaction times and higher standard deviations were found in data from women groups. The sex-related differences were found to increase over time. The relation of simple reaction performance to age and sex tends to be essentially the same as for choice reaction performance. A distinct difference between the simple and complex reaction times became evident, however, inasmuch as they are not equally trainable and training effects are not equally long-lasting. Whereas considerable training effects became evident for choice reaction performance, they could not be established for simple reaction performance. Observable improvement in simple reaction performance was limited to the early stages of practice, which in our study took place during the pretest. Subsequent training experience was not accompanied by performance improvement.

Other differences between choice reaction performance and simple reaction concern the conditions under which reaction performance was found to differ, and the variables found to influence reaction speed. For simple reaction performance in particular, specifically functional considerations played an important role, in which speed and visual components could be differentiated. This is indicated directly by the observed relation to eyesight and indirectly by other findings, such as the existence of a positive correlation for reaction speed following visual but not acoustic signals and the partial correlation to intelligence pertaining only to the HAWIE performance subtests. Since these connections are so consistently limited to specifically functional aspects, the use of simple reaction speed as an indicator variable yielding information on the functional status of the underlying perceptive system and, consequently, the central nervous system seems quite plausible. An important influence on the functional status of the perceptive system can be seen in a further specialized aspect, blood supply as related to circulation. It seems highly probable that blood supply, dependent on adequate circulation in the brain, has an effect on the specialized and highly sensitive functioning represented by simple reaction speed.

Comprehensive Interpretation and Conclusions of the Results on Psychomotor Performance and Reaction Time in Old Age

The two reaction performance types investigated in this study resemble each other in that both appear to be sensitive to influences of age and sex, with sex differences favoring the men in both functional areas. Critical reflection of the results soon makes it clear, however, that age is by no means the sole dominant influence. Rather, the performance ability in both functional areas seems to be codetermined by a great number of other variables which are essentially not confined to the central nervous system. The nature of these influencing variables, however, is quite different for the two types of performance investigated in this study. For one thing there are differences in the degree of lasting training effects. Whereas considerable training effects are found for necessarily more complex choice reaction performance, there are no training effects to speak of on simple reaction performance. In the latter, there was only a slight improvement in performance at the beginning of training and it seems to be largely the result of purely functional exercise. Further essential differences between the two functions can be summarized as follows. As might be expected, the nature of psychological, physical, and social influences on the more complex choice reaction task are rather complex. Major importance can be ascribed to general physical status, subjective feeling of physical well-being and relative freedom from physical problems, formal education, occupation, social status, intelligence, and general personal activity. The results of psychomotor choice reaction measurements seem to reflect a component of general flexibility and general drive in addition to a component of general physical health. By the same token, the results of choice reaction experiments seem to be appropriate indicator variables for the above mentioned psychophysical capacities.

The findings on important variables influencing simple reaction speed create quite a different picture. Here we find a much more predominant, strictly functional aspect, consisting primarily of a visual functional relation and a speed component. A much closer relation to central nervous system functioning, therefore, seems likely in the case of simple reaction performance. Another narrowly defined influence variable seems to be the general blood supply and circulation, particularly in the brain. From the standpoint of prophylactic geriatrics, our results emphasize the importance not only of maintaining adequate physical functioning but of actively encouraging the development of flexibility and activity in mental functioning. To a certain degree, challenges should remain part of the way of life on into old age. This is particularly true for intellectual life, for example accepting new responsibilities, where certain demands must be met and goals can be individually defined. Of course, the results indicate that exorbitant demands, overly ambitious goals, and hectic activity are not beneficial. Women seem to find increased social involvement particularly meaningful, especially when it extends beyond the immediate family. Positive acceptance of the general life situation and a feeling of being needed seems to be especially important. Considering the importance of these general drive and training factors and their ability to influence or retard the process of aging, the relative importance of chronological age is diminished. Psychomotor or sensorimotor age, largely a matter of vitally important flexibility, activity and general performance tendencies, is different from chronological age, as can be seen from the high variability of performance of elderly subjects.

On the other hand, we can describe something like 'functional age' on the basis of our results on simple reaction speed. Simple reaction speed seems to be an important index of functional age. Our results show that functional age is not identical to chronological age. Furthermore, it seems to be independent of a presumably inevitable, developmentally determined 'primary process of aging' in the neurophysiological sense described by *Birren.* The related factors of blood supply and circulation appear to have a major influence on functional age, and should accordingly be a major target of prophylactic and therapeutic geriatric efforts.

Psychomotor and functional age can serve as important indicators of age in a broad sense, meaning the capacity to perform in essential and basic life functions and activities, independent of chronological age. Thus, they are relevant measures, and they can generally be assessed without difficulty.

Contr. hum. Dev., vol. 3, pp. 51–67 (Karger, Basel 1976)

V. Consistency and Change of Personality Variables in Late Life

Heinz H. Grombach

Introduction

In the studies of the *Arbeitsgruppe Alternsforschung Bonn* (1971) (Bonn Gerontological Research Team), both cross-sectional and longitudinal analyses indicated that intellectual variables should not be studied without reference to other personality variables. *Lehr* (1967) and *Schreiner* (1969, 1970a-c, 1971a, b) underlined the significance of the outlook toward the future for a characterization of the present biographical situation. Not only were directly proportional relationships found between attitude toward the future and intellectual capacity, in addition, *Schreiner* (1970c, p. 282) discovered 'that disturbance or balance in certain areas of life together with increased attention to these conditions lead older persons to direct their thoughts about the future primarily to the areas in question'. Contrary to the assumption that aged persons' attitude toward the future is largely determined by the approaching of life with a consequently narrower range and more negative shading (*Buehler,* 1959; *Cumming and Henry,* 1961; *Moers,* 1953; *Stern,* 1955; *Vischer,* 1949), most experimental studies come to the conclusion 'that a drop and negative shading in attitudes toward the future depend on social and personality factors as well as the experience of the present life situation' (*Fink,* 1957; *Tuckman and Lorge,* 1954; *Feifel,* 1957; *Shelton and Kogan,* 1962; *Kastenbaum and Durkee,* 1964; *Schreiner,* 1970a-c).

Longitudinal empirical results about the thematic analysis of personality based on questions as to the extent and conditions of changes in 'life themes' or 'themes of existence' are far underrepresented in the literature. Theoretical limitations have contributed to this oversight in so far as most longitudinal studies are confined to narrowly circumscribed behavior aspects. Methodological difficulties (criteria for reliability and validity, scaling problems, etc.) are also practically responsible for this research deficit. However, some cross-cultural evidence

(*Puschner,* 1968; *Puschner et al.,* 1968) indicates that an increase of restrictive themes in old age is not generally the rule. The total biographical situation was found to have a greater effect on extending the relation to the future (desire to widen fields of interest, etc.) than chronological age. *Tismer* (1970) observed an unflagging desire for 'experiential opportunities' and for 'taking part in what's happening' among subjects in their seventies and eighties. In 1969, *Tismer* stated as a main conclusion 'that criteria such as age, social status, intelligence, and health status are of relatively little significance in respect to themes of existence, whereas variables more closely related to meaningful experiences and current social activity together with certain formal personality characteristics clearly contribute to the predominance of certain themes of conduct observed in our study' (p. 204). A more detailed consideration of the interaction of these variables over time follows in the discussion. Further German contributions to the discussion of this and related topics can be found in publications by *Thomae* (1968a, b), *Opgenoorth and Thomae* (1970), *Opgenoorth* (1971), *Thomae and Lehr* (1968) and *Lehr* (1972).

At this point we shall report briefly on selected findings dealing with consistency and change of behavioral categories such as activity, mood, etc., and findings on rigidity in advancing age as investigated in the present study and in *Angleitner's* contribution (chap. VI). In both the Duke Longitudinal Study (*Palmore,* 1970, 1974a, b; *Maddox,* 1963, 1965) and the Bethesda Longitudinal Study, (*Birren et al.,* 1963a, b; *Singer,* 1968), only small changes of activity in old age were found. According to *Youmans* and *Yarrow* (1969), changes of (social) activity and changes in the scope of interests are less related to changes in a person's own health than to intensely experienced events such as losing a loved one in old age. The relations between activity and mood on contentment are frequently discussed in connection with problems of 'disengagement' (*Maddox,* 1965; *Lehr,* 1972; *Neugarten,* 1973). *Maddox and Eisdorfer* (1963, p. 244) found that for the greater part of their sample the combination 'positive state of mood under the lack of high activity' did not occur, and 'negative "mood" proved to be usually connected with lower activity'. The authors add that the subjective rating of activity by the individual is of great importance.

Cross-sectional results of the BLSA indicate that activity, mood, ego control and self-confidence are to be explained less by age than by 'syndromes' of personality variables (state of health, rigidity, intolerance) and by 'destiny' (education, profession, social status; *Simons et al.,* 1968, p. 221; *Lehr and Rudinger,* 1969). Results from longitudinal analyses (*Rudinger and Feger,* 1970; *Rudinger and Erlemeier,* 1970; *Grombach,* 1973) are summarized in a passage below.

For a long time, rigidity, as a measure of lacking flexibility, directly corresponded to one of the most frequent assumptions about personality change in late life. However, factor-analytic studies have since established the necessity of distinguishing between different kinds of rigidity which relate to personality dimensions (drive level, neuroticism, etc.; *Brengelmann* and *Brengelmann,* 1960a, b; *Holland,* 1964), age, and intelligence (*Schaie,* 1958; *Luchins and Luchins,* 1959; *Riegel and Riegel,* 1960; *Chown,* 1961; *Heron and Chown,* 1967; *Erlemeier and Angleitner,* 1971).

Whereas significant age correlations (cross-sectional) were found for scales measuring rigidity, dogmatism, and attitude toward life (present and future and past) especially by *Riegel and Riegel* (1960) using the questionnaire they constructed, longitudinal results of the BLSA indicate that 'over a period of five years the distinction of rigid, dogmatic attitudes of aged persons as well as attitude toward the past, present, and future remain rather constant' (*Angleitner,* 1974a, b).

Consistency and Variability of Personality Characteristics in the Bonn Longitudinal Study of Aging

Grombach's (1973, 1975) longitudinal analyses follow the lines set by the BLSA concepts and the views of personality in works by *Cattell* (1965), *Thomae* (1968a-d), and *Herrmann* (1969, 1973). They include T, Q and L data as described extensively in other publications (*Thomae et al.,* 1973; *Grombach,* 1975; *Rudinger,* this volume, chap. III). The present description of these longitudinal results will concentrate on the discussion of intra- and interindividual constancy, and variability of the L data (*Thomae,* chap. I and XII). This representation will be extended by a short summary of results for the T and Q data.

The analyses are based on data from the longitudinal sample at measurement points I (1965/66), III (1967/68), and IV (1969/70). As far as sex- or cohort-specific influences on consistency or variability of intra- or interindividual differences were found, they will be reported separately. Otherwise the representation of the results refers to the entire sample. An extensive reproduction of the tables would take more space than is available here, but complete information is obtainable from the author (cf. *Grombach,* 1975).

The statistical analysis makes use of both descriptive and correlative techniques as well as factor-analytic and analysis of variance methods (*Rudinger,* chap. III), with combinations of the latter (e.g. generalization study with the factors of 'formal aspects of behavior').

Estimates of Corrected Reliability and Stability Coefficients for the Total Group

Following *Coleman*'s (1968) path analysis considerations, the estimates of corrected reliability and stability coefficients were computed and interpreted in accordance with *Heise*'s (1972) formulas and instructions. The assumptions and restrictions involved must be kept in mind, especially in relation to the influence

Table I. Estimates of corrected reliability and stability coefficients[1] for the total group (*Heise*, 1972)

Variables	Reliability coefficient	Stability coefficients		
	rxx	s I/III	s III/IV	s I/IV
Number of persons in the household	0.75	1.00 st	0.99 st	1.00 st
Subjective estimation of health	0.41	0.74 st	1.00 st	0.82 st
Attitude to other people	0.56	1.00 st	0.91 st	0.90 st
Feeling needed by others	0.88	0.62	0.67	0.42
Extension of plans	0.20	0.83 st	1.00 st	1.00 st
Satisfaction with present life situation	–0.15	–0.26 st	–1.00 st	0.90 st
Hawie (in English WAIS)				
Score on verbal part	0.89	0.99 st	0.96 st	0.95 st
Score on nonverbal part	0.85	0.92 st	1.00 st	0.96 st
Total score	0.94	0.95 st	0.99 st	0.94 st
Riegel				
General rigidity	0.70	0.90 st	0.99 st	0.89 st
Personal rigidity	0.65	0.99 st	1.00 st	1.00 st
Intolerance	0.54	0.80 st	0.85 st	0.68 st
Dogmatism	0.65	0.86 st	0.97 st	0.83 st
Attitude to future and past	0.57	0.88 st	1.00 st	0.88 st
Attitude to the present	0.75	0.81 st	0.84 st	0.68
Behavior Ratings (formal aspects of behavior)				
Activity	0.83	0.87 st	0.84 st	0.73
Kind of activity	0.68	0.95 st	0.99 st	0.94 st
Mood	0.58	0.65 st	0.70 st	0.46
General responsiveness	0.65	0.93 st	0.99 st	0.92 st
Adjustment	0.43	0.94 st	1.00 st	1.00 st
Ego control	0.76	0.66	0.58	0.38
Self-confidence	0.42	1.00 st	1.00 st	1.00 st
Health status (physician)	0.46	1.00 st	0.66 st	0.82 st
Basic concerns (content aspects of behavior)				
Initiative and resourcefulness	0.66	0.54	0.89 st	0.48
Impact of disappointments	0.45	0.91 st	1.00 st	0.95 st
Coming to terms with past fate	1.00	0.31	0.41	0.13
Coping with life's transience	0.35	0.65 st	0.82 st	0.53 st
Religious involvement	0.68	0.90 st	0.96 st	0.87 st
Widening the scope of interests	0.27	0.76 st	1.00 st	1.00 st
Maintaining social contacts	–0.08	–0.01	–1.00 st	0.07

of correlated errors in measurement. *Heise* himself included examples to demonstrate how ambiguity in measurement can affect stability coefficients. For example, if the stability coefficients of neighboring measurement points (say, s I/II and s II/III) are higher than the corrected reliability coefficient rxx whereas the stability coefficient s I/III is not, then this 'instability' is attributed to errors in measurement. However, a more detailed method of separation is not given by *Heise*. Table I presents all corrected reliability and stability coefficients.

Four variables have reliability coefficients which are strikingly lower than the rest. They are the extent of plans, contentment with the present, orientation toward widening the scope of interests, and efforts to maintain social contacts. All other variables show reliability coefficients of at least 0.35 or 0.42. As was to be expected, the corrected reliability coefficients shifted more or less after the addition of a third measurement point.

Since the results for men and women do not differ substantially, we can briefly point out the characteristics which underwent an observable change over the 5-year period of investigation for the sample as a whole. The stability coefficients reveal changes particularly for the variables 'feeling needed', 'self-control', 'initiative and resourcefulness', 'coming to terms with past fate' and efforts toward 'widening the scope of social contacts', and 'maintaining social contacts'. Except for the indications of low stability of 'self-control', these results are largely in agreement with previous information. Consequently, changes in T and Q data are more rare than changes in themes of existence and other L data obtained from interviews.

These results contributed to the decision to undertake a separate factor analysis followed by a stability and generalizability study of the behavior ratings which included two measures with unclear stability (amount of activity, mood) and one measure whose low stability indicated change (self-control). This constellation was judged to be the one most adequately fulfilling the requirements for such an analysis.

Factor-Analytic Studies of the Personality Characteristics for the Whole Sample over Several Measurement Points

Detailed descriptions of the computational procedures are given in other publications (*Thomae et al.,* 1973; *Grombach,* 1973, 1975; *Rudinger,* this volume, chap. III). The applied criteria yielded five factors for each point of measurement.

---

1 In cases where the stability coefficients turn out to be higher than the estimated reliability – indicating relative stability of the characteristic over a 5-year period of research – this is marked by 'st'.

Factor 1 of the 1965/66 measurement point covers social and activity-related variables. It remains stable in the years 1967/68 (where it becomes factor 2). In 1969/70, it includes all the characteristics of the formal aspects of behavior considered in this study. A more detailed longitudinal analysis of these characteristics follows below. The global measures of themes of existence in the years 1965/66 reoccur in the comparable factor 2. The variables loading on this factor are efforts expended toward coming to terms with past fate, coping with life's transience, and expanding the scope of social contacts and interests. We can say that this factor emphasizes basic themes in the biography of the individual.

In the first test-free interval, which lasted till the second measurement point in 1967/68, this factor already begins differentiating into one aspect composed of impact of disappointments, attitude toward future and past, and another pertaining to coming to terms with past fate and coping with life's transience (1967/68: factor 1).

Factor 5 of the years 1967/68 later extends into the area of social and religious involvement in 1967/68. In addition to the original variables 'attitude toward others', 'feeling needed', and 'satisfaction with present life situation' (which we shall consider later as a measure of 'inner balance' in our discussion of adjustment), the social and religious components join this factor in 1967/68.

During the next test-free interval, the themes of existence and assessments of the present just discussed underwent further changes before the 1969/70 measurement session. In some respects they parallel the trends from 1967/68, but unsystematic variations in the factor loadings are also observable. For example, in the years 1969/70 factor 5 contains only (negative loading) variables pertaining to expansive orientation in the fields of social relations and outside interests.

Throughout the entire period of investigation, factor 3 lends itself to interpretation as a dimension of rigidity-flexibility. Whereas in 1965/66 only questionnaire data load negatively on factor 3, a bipolar factor follows in 1969/70, lending support to the conclusion that relations do exist between higher scale values on rigidity measures, lower intellectual achievement on IQ tests, and less extensive plans for the near future.

Measures of 'intentional behavior control' and the physician's assessment of health remain in factor 4 from 1965/66 to 1967/68. In the interval before 1969/70, 'adjustment' and 'ego control' join the other formal aspects of behavior, as mentioned above. In their place, variables concerning themes of existence become evident.

The subsequent similarity rotations were carried out to clarify the nature of the stability or instability of the factor structures and variables over the 5-year period of investigation. Rotations of the factor solutions and similarity coefficients of the factor matrices, factors, and variables under comparison were calculated using the procedures developed by *Sixtl* (1964) and *Fischer and Roppert*

(1964). Only for adjacent measurement points could sufficient similarity (0.79–0.84) be confirmed. Similarity coefficients between 1965/66 and 1969/70 do not meet the 0.80 criterion (they do, however, reach 0.72).

Four variables had insufficient similarity coefficients for all three measurement points. These variables, which showed evidence of clear changes in their relationships to the other variables, were 'extent of plans', 'maintaining social contacts', and the two formal behavior characteristics 'adjustment' and 'self-control'. It should be kept in mind, in this context, that reliabilities of estimates concerning the extent of plans and efforts to preserve social contact were not high enough. Judging by *Simons et al.* (1968) and our own results, this is not necessarily the case for the formal behavior aspects.

Further computations served to verify these results. The formal variables of behavior were factor-analyzed with subsequent generalizability studies. In addition, analyses of variance were calculated for all characteristics for repeated measurements with different independent variables.

Results of the Generalizability Study

The criteria of extraction suggest a two-factor solution for the formal aspects of behavior. At all measurement points, factor 1 includes the variables 'extent of activity', 'mood', 'kind of activity', and 'self-confidence'. Factor 2 consists of 'adjustment' and 'ego control'. These factor structures can be compared to results obtained with similar behavior ratings for other samples (*Thomae,* 1968a-d). Doing so leads us to interpret factor 1 as a 'social and achievement activity' dimension and factor 2 as an 'intentional behavior control' dimension.

The similarity coefficients turned out to be extremely high for both men and women. This holds for both factors and all measurement point comparisons (table II). The similarity coefficients vary (over the measurement points I, III, and IV) from 0.96 to 0.99. Even the only exception, the variable 'mood', reaches the 0.80 criterion. The stability of the two dimensions was verified according to *Heise* (1972), with the results as shown in table III.

The 'social and achievement activity' dimension seems to be rather stable for both men and women. The reliability and stability coefficients hardly differ, even over the entire 5-year period of observation. We can therefore conclude that, for the first dimension, extensive intra- and interindividual changes over the observed measurement period are not likely in our sample.

The assumption of changes in the 'intentional behavior control'dimension in the course of the study is more likely. Remarkable differences of the coefficients were found for the period between 1965/66 and 1969/70, although differences between adjacent measurement points were not so striking. In our sample, intentional behavioral control appears to have undergone rather extensive change over a period of 5 years.

Table II. Similarity coefficients of both factors over three measurement points for the entire sample

	Measurement point			
	I		III	
	factor 1	factor 2	factor 1	factor 2
Measurement point III				
Factor 1	0.99			
Factor 2		0.99		
Measurement point IV				
Factor 1	0.98		0.99	
Factor 2		0.95		0.98

Table III. Corrected reliability and stability coefficients over three measurement points

Coefficients	Factors	
	1	2
Corrected reliability		
$r_{I/III}$	0.69	0.59
$r_{III/IV}$	0.74	0.51
$r_{I/IV}$	0.63	0.43
r_{xx}	0.81	0.70
Stability		
$s_{I/III}$	0.85	0.79
$s_{III/IV}$	0.91	0.68
$s_{I/IV}$	0.79	0.63

Table IV. Components of variance (CV) and percentage of the components of variance in the generalizability study

	Men				Women			
	factor 1		factor 2		factor 1		factor 2	
	CV	%	CV	%	CV	%	CV	%
Ss	0.06	5.7	0.08	6.0	0.26	20.1	0.29	23.2
Scales	0.08	6.7	0.08	6.3	0.07	5.5	0.08	6.1
Time	−0.01	−0.1	0.01	00.1	−0.02	−0.1	0.02	0.2
Ss scales	0.4	34.9	0.5	38.9	0.41	32.2	0.43	36.1
Ss x time	0.07	5.7	0.08	6.8	0.05	4.0	0.05	4.2
Scales x time	0.01	0.9	0.02	1.7	0.02	1.5	0.02	1.6
Residual	0.5	46.2	0.42	34.6	0.46	36.7	0.40	31.7

Table V. Generalizability coefficients

Universe	Men		Women	
	factor 1	factor 2	factor 1	factor 2
Time and scales (random)	0.39	0.42	0.72	0.58
Time	0.72	0.70	0.89	0.76
Scales (fixed)	0.51	0.52	0.77	0.72

A generalizability study was conducted for the dimensions 'social and achievement activity' and 'intentional behavior control' in the light of the methodological considerations mentioned above. The results of these calculations for men and women are contrasted in table IV.

The residual variance constitues the largest component of variance in factor 1, due primarily to triple interactions and measurement error. Nonetheless, the satisfactory reliability coefficients allow interpretation of the results. We find only one notable main effect. In the subsample of women, it occurs in factors 1 and 2 in the form of components of variance due to subjects. The components of variance for interactions between subjects and scales (averaged over three measurement points) are all high. The percentage fluctuates between 32 and 39%. These interactions are indicative of different characteristic profiles over time. The results show that the main effects, 'time', 'scales', and 'scales x time' interaction, all have only minor components of variance. As a result, we can expect the basic data pool to provide information on longitudinal trends only under the condition that interindividual differences are taken into account in subsequent analyses. This condition is further supported by the components of variance related to the main effect 'subjects', especially in the women of our sample. We can assume a certain generalizability of these results to be possible, especially if time or scales are treated as fixed factors (table V).

On the basis of these results it becomes necessary to investigate the possibility of interindividual differences in the development of the formal behavior aspects rated in our study. This will be attempted below, together with a consideration of possible determinants.

Results of the Analyses of Variance for Repeated Measurements and Constancy and Variability of Personality Variables

A look at the variance tables from various analyses (*Grombach,* 1975) reveals that the influence of the independent variables 'age' (cohorts) and 'time' (measurement points) has rather narrow limits. The results can be briefly summarized as follows.

Influences of Age and Time

Age and time have very little effect on the behavior ratings in our sample (factor 1): Eta % lies between 0.07 and 2.22. On the one hand, these characteristics appear to be rather constant, but, by the same token, no corresponding differences can be found between cohorts. A significant main effect for time was found in factor 2, which includes various health measures in addition to variables concerning attitudes and adjustment. However, chronological age accounts for only negligible variance in respect to the aspect of 'contentment with present situation' in this variable. By no means can we identify any notable effects upon the development of attitudinal variables which can be attributed to age. The main effect 'time' tends to significant values in other respects, namely subjectively experienced health problems and impact of disappointments. We also find no significantly different developments between different cohorts within dimension 3, which includes intelligence and rigidity variables together with a measure of time perspective. In respect to the extent of planes, 21% of the variance is accounted for by the main effect 'time'. However, this variable's reliability prevents us from placing too much weight on this finding.

The results for themes of existence (factor 4) present a similar picture. Whereas the main effect 'time' is responsible for approximately 11% of the variance for 'initiative and resourcefulness' and 34% for 'maintaining social contacts', the possibility of effects due to age is limited to the variable 'religious involvement'. Here, the older persons were consistently more involved throughout the period from 1965/66 to 1969/70. Finally, the theme of expansion, as it is encountered in factor 5, also shows little indication of being influenced by 'age'. Only the familiar effect of 'time' accounts for 11% of the variance for 'widening the scope of interests' and 62% of the variance for 'widening the scope of social contacts'. As pointed out earlier, the observed decrease in efforts to widen the scope of social contacts in both cohorts can be attributed to significant increases in efforts to maintain existing social contacts.

Effect of Socioeconomic Status, Time, and
Subjectively Experienced Health on the Dependent Variables

Significant relations of independent variables to the behavioral ratings (factor 1) are discernible only between socioeconomic status, extent of activity, general responsiveness and control. No interactions occurred between socioeconomic status, subjectively experienced health, and time.

These main effects of socioeconomic status on certain behavioral variables can be verified for all three measurement points and appear to be sex-specific. Among the men, socioeconomic status is responsible for 12–13% of the variance for 'ego control' compared to 2% among the women. Social status furthermore accounts for 15% of the variance in 'extent of activity' and 17% in ,responsiveness' in the group of women, compared to around 1 and 2, respectively, among the men. Obviously, social status influences the control of behavior to a greater extent among men than among women. Just the opposite seems to apply to the extent of activity and general responsiveness.

The second factor (attitude variables) follows the same general pattern. Social status can be observed to affect the kind of attitude toward others only among the women, where it accounts for 8% of the variance. The same holds for coming to terms with past fate (approximately 5% of the variance). However, 5% of this particular variance is related to the subjectively experienced state of health among both men and women. Among women, we find a significant interaction between social status and subjectively experienced health problems (12%). Interpretation of this last interaction is made difficult by the smaller sums of cells. This is also the case for significant triple interactions in regard to satisfaction with the present situation.

As anticipated, social status accounts for a high percentage of the total variance on HAWIE (factor 3). For men it repeatedly reaches the 24-percent level from 1965–66 to 1969/70; for women it remains steady at about 18%. We may add that knowledge of social status reduces the total variance (measurement points I–IV) of the verbal IQ about 23–25% for both men and women. It reduces the variance of the performance IQ about 16 and 14% for men and only about 7 or 5% (not significant) for women. There is no evidence of contrary developmental tendencies over the 5-year period of investigation, not even for differences in intellectual achievement on the HAWIE characterizing groups of differing socioeconomic status. Interactions between social status and time hover around zero.

Just as the total variance of the rigidity scales is reduced by knowlegde of social status, so, too, is the total variance of the variable 'widening the space of interests' (factor 5). The percentage of variance for the scales 'general' and 'personal' rigidity runs up to 8 and 11% across all measurement points for men and women.

Among men, social status is responsible for 11% of the observed variance for the variable 'widening the scope of interests', and among women it accounts for about 17% with minimal wavering over time.

Summing up, we can say that social status sheds considerable light on the total variance of a number of variables. In contrast, the amounts of variance due to the subjectively rated state of health are surprisingly small. In only one case did it reach a significant level (i.e. for coming to terms with past fate).

Interactions between both independent variables in relation to 'satisfaction with current life situation' in the course of time come closest to a reversal of this development trend.

Effect of Socioeconomic Status, Time, and General State of Health on the Dependent Variables

Additional main effects and interactions for general health status are presented below.

Two main effects of this independent variable are confined to the group of men. General health status, as rated by a physician, rather consistently accounts for around 10% of the total variance over time in respect to adjustment among men (women: 0.2%) and around 9% of the total variance for impact of disappointments (women: unter 1%). Among men, an additional 6–7% of the total variance for impact of disappointments are due to interactions between social status and general health status.

For women, 9–10% of the total variance for 'religious involvement' are explained by an interaction between these same variables, social status and general health status.

General health was found not to have any significant influence on variables dealing with activity and efforts toward personal expansion (e.g. widening the scope of interests). For the total sample, differences emerging with time in intellectual achievement on verbal HAWIE subtests can be explained to about 10% by the general state of health. Reactions of the whole sample on a stress reaction test are explained to about 7% by general health. This result obviously points to differences in health, as defined by *Birren* (1962), to be found among our subjects from 1965/66 to 1969/70.

Effect of Contentment with Present Life Situation and Extent of Plans

'Contentment with present life situation' and 'extent of plans' have hardly any part in main effects and interactions. They apparently fail to differentiate clearly for the greater part of our dependent variables. Among women, we find contentment with present life situation as a main effect (10–11% of the total variance) with regard to subjectively estimated health status and variables of time perspective in the Riegel questionnaire (attitudes toward present and toward future: 7–9% of the total variance). According to this finding, contentment with the present life situation is able to explain a certain amount of the total variance for other subjective ratings of stress situations and outlook on the present and future.

Comprehensive Discussion

Within the 5-year period of investigation, the least evidence of change was found for test and questionnaire data from our subjects. Both intellectual and psychomotor performance remain stable between 1965/66 and 1969/70. The same holds for the personality variables 'rigidity', 'dogmatism', 'attitude toward the past and future', and 'attitude toward the present'. As in other investigations (*Rudinger,* chap. III; *Angleitner,* chap. VI), changes due to aging are overshadowed by unchanging age-related differences. This emphasizes the previously mentioned advisability of treating behavioral development as more than just a function of 'growing old' (*Baer,* 1970, 1973; *Wohlwill,* 1970). 'The number of years which the individual has lived through is by no means the only or even the predominant factor involved in mental capacity' (*Lehr,* 1972). The view that chronologic 'age is at best an abbreviation for a multitude of events which have taken place and contributed their part to behavior changes' (*Rudinger,* 1971a-c) underlines the importance of understanding the aging process as a 'multidimensional structure of change' (*Thomae,* 1968a).

The possibility that asynchronous structures should appear in aging processes, documented by *Thomae* in concrete terms, does not contradict the multivariate determinants of personality. For example, *Thomae* (1968b, 1972) himself refers to social status as a 'socialization variable' with relevance for areas ranging from psychofunctional processes to matters of 'social competence'. This orientation is plain in other works, too. For example, *Thomae* 1970 outlines a cognitive personality theory of aging, wherein complex networks of relationships that include features of the subjective point of view are examined with a searching intensity seldom matched in the literature.

Measures of health as rated by a physician and the subjective estimate of health problems seem reliable enough and relatively stable between the years 1965/66 and 1969/70 in our longitudinal study (but compare *Lehr and Schmitz-Scherzer,* chap. XI). This is also the case for the overall impression rating score. Results of the generalizability studies for the factors 'social and achievement activity' and 'intentional control of behavior' suggested that only the findings on interindividual differences could be interpreted meaningfully.

The personality characteristics assessed by means of interviews present a more heterogeneous picture. The definition of the characteristics themselves, calculation of the stability coefficients, and analyses of variance allow us to differentiate between two groups of variables. Ample evidence points to the absence of marked change over the 5-year period of observation for the variables 'attitude toward others', 'impact of disappointments', 'coping with life's transience', 'coming to terms with past fate', 'widening the scope of interests', and 'religious involvement'. For a few other variables, however, the problems associated with errors in measurement (problem of reliability) and true changes remain.

The observed shift of emphasis from extending to maintaining social contacts are actually quite plausible. With growing age, concern with maintaining social contacts predominates over concern with widening their range, at least in our sample. The low reliability coefficients for the rating of 'maintaining', however, give rise to the objection that the background information related to behavior in interviews on topics of this nature changes freely over the years. It is therefore susceptible to being influenced by repeated measurement.

The influence of methodological procedures on results can be seen in the factor-analytic results, verified in like manner for both sexes, and most particulary in the similarity of factor matrices obtained for adjacent measurement points. Only the factors 'rigidity-flexibility' and 'activity' showed no significant changes in their structure within 5 years. This is bound to affect our conclusions about the constancy and variability of personality in old age. The longer the period of investigation, the more likely are structural changes in L data to be observed.

Since the greater likelihood of changes in longer intervals of time has been utilized in some models for investigating the process of psychological development (*Cattell,* 1970), the conclusion that these changes are not merely the result of errors in measurement can be justified.

Conditions for estabilishing a 'cognitive identity of the investigation situation', on the other hand, are somewhat less favorable for interview data. Repeated discussion on certain topics (e. g. social contacts, interests, religion) may very well have a habituating effect, diminishing the impact of emotional aspects on these topics by the third interview as compared to the first interview. Some variables cannot be completely freed of methodological artefacts.

To be sure, these flaws can be subsequently located, given the conditions characteristic of intensive longitudinal study, as described above. Measurement errors are all the less likely in cases where variables of this sort have rising scores.

Moreover, a number of changes in variables related to the subjective point of view, regardless whether they are 'methodological artefacts' or not, nonetheless reflect real developments and connections. For instance, less and less frequent mention of health problems, disappointments, and restrictions combined with active efforts to change the situations seem to function as a means of defending a particular self-concept which, for all its changeability, remains oriented toward the norms dictated by youth-centered values (*Theissen,* 1970a, b). Thus, changes in these ratings also relate to 'real' characteristics, which need only be critically evaluated in terms of their representativeness for the everyday behavior of our subjects (*Thomae et al.,* 1973).

It is interesting to note in this context that our subjects described themselves as more satisfied with the present situation from 1965/66 to 1969/70. At the same time, a number of significant relations to other 'cognitive' characteristics were verified both in 1967/68 and in 1969/70: namely, high correlations for the variables 'mood' (+), 'impact of disappointments' (–), and 'coming to terms with past fate' (–) point to thematic consistency, and a complementary development can be seen in the steadily improved subjective view of health, more positive attitudes toward others, and more frequent use of available opportunities, which are signs of more successful coping with the present situation. A more positive attitude toward the future is linked to greater contentment. In this context we must refer to the increasing importance of the individual's 'objective' health and the problems often dealt with in longitudinal studies of 'survivors' and 'dropouts'. Social status is not a direct index of contentment with the present life situation, but the statement that 'social structure creates the conditions for both change and stability in adult life' (*Bedler,* 1968) is to be taken seriously. This relates to indications based on our results, too, that social status affects variables of activity, intelligence (flexibility, rigidity), and health on the one hand, and attitudes toward other people, e. g. interests and coming to terms with past fate on the other.

At the beginning of this chapter we discussed the relations between T and Q data which remain constant over the research period. Using different correlational methods, additional invariant connections to some biographic characteristics were found. At all measurement points, intellectual performance shows significant correlations to different behavior ratings, especially to extent of activity, general responsiveness, ego control, and self-confidence (*Thomae,* 1968b). These results lend support to the findings of cross-sectional studies (*Simons et al.,* 1968) and of longitudinal investigations (*Owens,* 1966; *Palmore,* 1970, 1974a, b). Higher intellectual ability, measures of activity and responsiveness, and more marked ego control are found in conjunction with throughout the study. But as we have shown on the basis of factor analyses and factor structure comparisons for formal aspects of behavior, measures of activity, responsiveness, etc. should be understood here as a global evaluation of 'social and achievement activity'. Concentrating on more strictly social aspects of activity (e. g. the activity-disengagement controversy), various other studies have found more distinct relations to general contentment with life (*Lehr and Rudinger,* 1970; *Havighurst et al.,* 1969).

Palmore and Luikart (1974), who chose multiple regression analysis as the methodological basis for their study, also found no direct connection between intellectual ability and general satisfaction with the present life situation. Their results correspond to our findings that intelligence, activity (defined in terms of social engagement) and health considerations were connected with measures of 'intentional behavior control'.

The parallels between the findings of *Palmore and Luikart* (1974) and our findings continue. In both cases we find a strong connection between subjective health evaluation (itself correlated to the physician's evaluation) and general contentment with the present life situation. 'Self-rated health was by far the strongest variable related to life satisfaction and it alone accounts for two-thirds or more of the explained variance in all groups analyzed. This seems to confirm the old adage, "your health is the most important thing" ' (*Palmore und Luikart,* 1974).

In fact, we find a relationship of reciprocal influence between contentment with the present life situation and intentional behavior control in both studies of aged persons: 'Persons believing that they control their lives may engage in life styles that provide more satisfaction and persons who have more satisfying experiences may develop a stronger belief that they control their lives' (*Palmore and Luikart,* 1974).

If we understand 'life satisfaction' as a general measure of adjustment to aging, i. e. a state of relative balance between the individual's cognitive structure and his manner of coping with the present, then the results gathered up to now lend themselves to integration in a 'cognitive personality theory of aging' (*Thomae,* 1971a, b). It is to be hoped that further variables can be added at a later point. As pointed out by *Thomae* (1974a, b), the concepts 'adjustment', 'well-being', and 'contentment with life' are already used practically synonymously in English-language research. 'Thus, the social gerontological meaning of adjustment should be defined as achieving a state of equilibrium between the needs of individuals and the demands or burdens placed upon them by their respective life situations' (*Thomae,* 1974a).

The satisfaction with the present situation in life as the expression of successful coping with a particular life situation represents as a complex process of biographically interdependent relations (e. g. between social status, intellectual capacity, flexibility-rigidity, state of health) and their alternating effects on (cognitive) components of the subjective life space (time perspective, impact of disappointments, subjective rating of the state of health, attitude toward other people, coming to terms with past fate, interest, and so on). Inasmuch as the aging persons, who repeatedly placed themselves at our disposal for extensive observations from 1965 on, succeeded for the most part in handling their individual situation more and more successfully and in experiencing it as more and more satisfactory, we can conclude that the picture 'which we found in this study of the aged person is the picture of the 60-80-year-olds who feel accepted by a young research team and feel they are being taken seriously. In this sense, it is the picture of the aged person that would be representative for a society which knew how to integrate the aged. The validity of our conclusions therefore should not be determined in relation to the actual behavior of our subjects. Some of our results simply show, what could be the case for many older people' (cf. *Thomae et al.*, 1973). We can second the observation made by *Thomae* (1974a) that the concept of adjustment usually encountered in geropsychology and sociology can be smoothly integrated into physiological models of homeostasis (cf. *Keidel*, on certain cybernetic models).

In closing we can note from the theoretical point of view that by making use of longitudinal information on wider aspects of behavior the study succeeded in showing a complex system of conditions and interrelationships involved in the development of human behavior and experience. Studies of constancy and variability of personality among adults and aged persons are particularly well suited to help us understand the process of human development as a process of continuous adaptation. *Klausner* (1971) calls the process of 'adaptation' the most important dynamic concept in human ecology. 'Adaptation is both a key concept in ecology and key concept in the aging process . . . the aging process itself can be seen as one of continual adaptation: adaptation both to the external environment and to the changes in internal capabilities and functioning which take place during the life cycle' (cf. *Lawton and Nahemow*, 1973). From this standpoint it should be investigated to what extent the concept of adaptation can be considered an integrating influence in developmental and personality models in psychology.

Contr. hum. Dev., vol. 3, pp. 68–80 (Karger, Basel 1976)

VI. Changes in Personality Observed in Questionnaire Data from the Riegel Questionnaire on Rigidity, Dogmatism, and Attitude toward Life

A. Angleitner

Introduction and Previous Research

A review of research on changes in attitudes during old age led *Riegel and Riegel* (1960) to the construction of their own attitude scales. The items were taken from *Hardesty* (1954), *Rokeach et al.* (1955) and *Burgess et al.* (1953), and from original item formulations, especially for the interest scales and the attitude toward life scales. The scales consisted of Likert-type items: 6 for general rigidity (R_1), 6 for personal rigidity (R_2), 3 for anxiety (D_3), 4 for intolerance (D_4), 6 for general dogmatism (D_5), 7 for pro- and retrospective attitude toward life (L_6), 7 for contemporaneous attitude toward life (L_7), and 14 interest items (I). The items were formulated in English as well as German. It should be noted that in the Bonn Longitudinal Study of Aging (BLSA) the anxiety scale (D_3) was not used, the interest (I) scales were administered only once, and the L_7 scale was modified by excluding the items: 'I feel very old' and 'I feel that no one cares what happens to me'. With the exception of the work by *Riegel* and associates, the studies reported on below were carried out with the shortened version of the questionnaire. A higher score in R_1, R_2, D_4, or D_5 means an increase in the respective attitudes and, due to a departure from *Riegel and Riegel*'s (1960) scoring method, a higher score in L_6 or L_7 is taken to mean a more positive orientation toward life in our studies.

Reliability and Stability Coefficients of the Riegel Scales

These coefficients, using a formula developed by *Heise* (1972), for the four measurement times of the BLSA are given in table I (*Schmitz-Scherzer,* 1975 c).

Although the results do not reveal the Riegel scales to be very precise and reliable measuring instruments, they are roughly comparable to the test-retest coefficients reported by *Riegel et al.* (1967). Factor analysis of the scales over three times of measurement yielded two factors: a rigidity factor (R_1, R_2, D_5) and an attitude toward life factor (L_6, L_7.) The intolerance scale D_4 just barely

Table I. Reliability and stability of the Riegel scales according to *Schmitz-Scherzer* (1975c)

Variable	Total		Men		Women	
	reliability	stability	reliability	stability	reliability	stability
Riegel R_1	0.694	0.880	0.681	0.908	0.715	0.852
Riegel R_2	0.701	0.762	0.671	0.846	0.730	0.673
Riegel D_4	0.454	0.461	0.693	0.342	0.214	0.912
Riegel D_5	0.650	0.575	0.491	0.949	0.932	0.277
Riegel L_6	0.661	0.524	0.623	0.620	0.626	0.612
Riegel L_7	0.692	0.604	0.768	0.934	0.613	0.725

met the communality requirements allowing for its interpretation as a rigidity factor. A factor structure comparison showed these two factors to be sufficiently similiar over a measurement period of 5 years (*Angleitner,* 1974a), and a study using the generalizability concept of *Gleser et al.* (1965) indicates that these results could be replicated for other measurement times (*Angleitner,* 1974b).

In the original analysis of the questionnaire in 1960, *Riegel and Riegel* suggested that single and combined scores could be used. By combined scores they mean the sums of the scale scores for R_1+R_2, D_4+D_5, and L_6+L_7. More recent results by *Angleitner* (1974a, b) suggest that it is not clear whether these scale pairs measure the same dimensions and it therefore does not seem justified to use the summation procedure.

Construct Validity of the Riegel Scales

There is also some information on the construct validity of the Riegel scales. The rigidity and dogmatism scales show significant correlations with other rigidity, dogmatism and intolerance scales constructed by *Brengelmann and Brengelmann* (1960a, b) as shown in table II. These correlations can be taken as evidence for sufficient construct validity of all but one (D_4) of the Riegel scales.

The finding of a negative relationship between rigidity and intelligence measurements has been reported by a number of authors in previous research (*Schaie,* 1958; *Brengelmann and Brengelmann,* 1960b; *Chown,* 1961) and gained new support from our results in respect to the Riegel scales. Our study showed that scales measuring rigidity or dogmatism correlated negatively with intelligence scores on verbal WAIS and Raven CPM (*Angleitner,* 1972). *Riegel et al.* (1962) found a similar relation between rigid attitudes and educational level.

For the scales L_6 and L_7 measuring attitude toward life and a rating scale of

Table II. Correlations between Brengelmann scales (NR = rigidity; DO = dogmatism; IA = intolerance) and Riegel scales (R_1, R_2, D_4, D_5)

Variable	Sample						
	70-year-old subjects (*Angleitner*, 1972)			80-year-old subjects (*Angleitner*, 1972)			BLSA
	NR	DO	IA	NR	DO	IA	NR
R_1	0.39	0.38	0.52	0.48	0.33	0.60	0.31
R_2	0.40	0.26	0.34	0.33	0.19	0.41	0.22
D_4	0.34	0.36	0.30	0.18	0.30	0.31	−0.03
D_5	0.31	0.41	0.38	0.29	0.36	0.35	0.23

Table III. Correlations of the Riegel scales with age

Sample	Scale					
	R_1	R_2	D_4	D_5	L_6	L_7
Riegel and Riegel (1960) 55- to 75-year-old and older subjects	0.19[1]	0.20[1]	0.08	0.06	0.20[1]	0.10[1]
BLSA 65- to 84-year-old subjects	0.12	0.12	0.14	0.23[1]	−0.08	−0.07
Angleitner (1972) 52- to 94-year-old subjects	0.15[1]	0.16[1]	0.05	0.25[1]	−0.28[1]	0.04

1 Significance at $p < 0.01$.

attitude toward the future based on personal interviews, a stable positive correlation was found. The correlations averaged 0.38 for L_6 and 0.29 for L_7 over four periods of measurement. The scales L_6 and L_7 also correlate negatively with the following series of measures: subjective health rating, state of health as rated by a physician, anxiety (MAS), and neuroticism (N from ENNR). As a group, persons who felt themselves to be in poor health as well as those with high anxiety and neuroticism scores had characteristically more negative attitudes toward life.

Research Findings with the Riegel Questionnaire

Cross-Sectional Studies

In their study, *Riegel and Riegel* (1960, p. 185) found 'a consistent rise in rigidity over the whole age span'. This increase was also more marked, especially for men, on those scales consisting of general stereotyped phrases, namely general rigidity (R_1) and general dogmatism (D_5). For scales with items formulated in the first person (R_2, D_3, D_4) this trend was not so marked. Their analyses also revealed a more negative attitude toward life (L_6, L_7) with advancing age, which was not quite regular, particularly among women. Higher scores were obtained by women on the interest scales. Women also exhibited a greater degree of anxiety (D_3) and intolerance (D_4) than men. Table III shows the correlations of the questionnaire scales with age as obtained in the studies by *Riegel and Riegel* (1960), *Angleitner* (1972), and from the present investigation of the BLSA sample.

The correlations between the rigidity and intolerance scales differ somewhat, with only the data from *Riegel and Riegel* (1960) and *Angleitner* (1972) indicating an increase in rigidity with advancing age. Further differences become evident in the D_5 and L_7 scales. The difference in sign for L_6 is an artifact produced by different scoring weights. In the BLSA sample, the endorsement of generally formulated dogmatism items (D_5) increased markedly with increasing age. The postulated negative attitude toward life could not be replicated with the BLSA.

In a multiple analysis of variance design with the treatments age, sex, and educational level, *Angleitner* (1972) found that compared to the younger age group (52–75 years), higher age (76–94 years) was accompanied by higher rigidity and dogmatism scores (R_1^{ss}, R_2^{s}, D_5^{ss}; s = significant at the $p < 0.05$ level, ss = significant at the $p < 0.01$ level) and a more negative attitude toward life on the L_6 scale in which, according to its authors, 'some expectancies about the future are expressed or in which the present is valued in terms of the past' (*Riegel and Riegel,* 1960, pp. 192–193). Educational level was associated with general rigidity (R_1^{ss}). Persons who finished high school or university-like institutions were much less inclined to endorse the generally phrased stereotyped R_1

sentences than others with incomplete secondary or advanced education. Men had higher scores in general rigidity ($R_1{}^s$) than women. However, by controlling health data and intellectual achievement, these effects were reducible.

In a study by *Erlemeier and Angleitner* (1971), comparing the BLSA sample with the financially and educationally better situated sample used by *Angleitner* (1972), it could be shown that the two samples differed most notably in intelligence as measured by the Raven CPM and on the scales R_1, R_2, and D_4. The longitudinal sample, seen as having lower socioeconomic status, could be described as more rigid and intolerant compared with the *Angleitner* (1972) sample with higher SES. The age effects over both samples are similiar to the findings of *Angleitner* described above. For men and women a difference was found on L_7, with men showing a more positive attitude toward life than women, i. e. more endorsement of 'statements on the subject's present feeling of acceptance, usefulness, and well-being' (*Riegel and Riegel,* 1960, p. 184).

Longitudinal Studies

After 5 years, 202 persons of the original sample (n = 380) used by *Riegel and Riegel* (1960) could be retested. 62 persons were deceased, 32 were too ill, and 84 refused to participate, as reported by *Riegel et al.* (1967). Various subgroup comparisons between the mean scores at the first testing of the original samples revealed that retested subjects 'represent biased samples'. Compared to the original group of participants as a whole and especially those not retested, subjects who returned for retesting are less rigid, slightly less dogmatic, and more positive in their attitudes toward life. In an analysis of cohort differences (persons grouped by birth dates in 5-year periods, e. g. 1897–1901, 1892–1896, etc.) and time differences between the first and second testing of retestees, *Riegel et al.* (1967) found significant cohort differences for the scales $R_1{}^s$, $R_2{}^s$, $D_5{}^{ss}$, $L_7{}^s$ and significant time differences for the scales $R_1{}^{ss}$, $R_2{}^{ss}$, and $L_7{}^{ss}$. Cohort x time interactions were established for $R_2{}^s$ and $D_5{}^s$. Higher age was associated with more rigidity and a more negative attitude toward life but with slightly less dogmatism than was to be expected on the basis of cross-sectional data. For the lower age levels, longitudinal trends closely matched the mean values from cross-sectional comparisons.

Topics for Investigation

Previous findings suggest the investigation of the following four points: (1) Over a period of 7 years, are longitudinal changes to be expected in measurements obtained from scales purporting to measure rigidity, dogmatism, attitude toward the present, and attitude toward the past and future? (2) Are such changes expected to occur to the same extent in groups with different socioeconomic status (upper versus lower) or sex? (3) Do observed differences persist when intellectual ability and state of health as diagnosed by a physician are controlled? (4) How do the present sample's scores on these scales compare with those of a control sample selected in a similar manner?

Methods, Subjects, and Procedures

Longitudinal Study

Data for this longitudinal study (computations with the Datatext program were performed on an IBM 360 at the 'Institut für Instrumentelle Mathematik', Friedrich-Wilhelm-Universität, Bonn) were obtained from 119 persons (63 men and 56 women) from the BLSA sample described in more detail in Chapter 2. In addition, a control sample of 27 men and 30 women, comparable to the longitudinal sample in age, sex, education, and other personal statistics, were tested at the last session in 1972/73. Measurement times for the longitudinal sample were in 1965/66, 1967/68, 1969/70, and 1972/73.

Shortened version of the Riegel Scales

Data were obtained from the shortened version of scales developed by *Riegel and Riegel* (1960). Additional data in this study are the summed raw scores on WAIS verbal subtests; a physician's rating of each subject's state of health, from 1 = excellent to 5 = very poor, and SES, taking an experimenter rating of 1–2 as low, 3 as medium and 4–5 as high.

Three-Way Analyses of Variance

Three-way analyses of variance were computed with the treatments (a) sex (masculine versus feminine); (b) SES (1–2 versus 3 versus 4–5); and (c) time (measurement points I–IV) as repeated factor. The age factor was deleted from this study, because it made the cell frequencies too small and unbalanced for computation. Preliminary four-way analyses of variance further justify this procedure, since no significant effects were produced by the age factor. We have used the 'fixed-effects' model approach here (*Hays,* 1973), which means that our generalizations are limited to the sample used. Taking the Riegel scales as independent variables, a three-factor analysis of variance was computed for each scale.

A check of the homogeneity of variances indicated that particulary for SES the variances were frequently most unhomogeneous. Computations were nevertheless considered justifiable due to the robustness of the F test in the fixed model (*Hays,* 1973). When the number of cases is not the same for all cells, the method of unweighted means applies; i. e., row and column means 'are simple means of the cell means regardless of the number of cases of the cells' (*Armor and Couch,* 1972, p. 113). As *Armor and Couch* (1972, p. 112) put it, this 'method results in approximations as long as the cell N-s are not too unequal (no more than a 4 to 1 ratio or so)'.

Finally, analyses of covariance were then carried out (*Winer,* 1971, pp. 605 ff.), with the covariates 'sum of all verbal WAIS subtest scores' and 'physician's rating of health'. The unequal cell numbers made a conclusive check of regression homogeneities impossible. Consequently, the results of the analyses of covariance should be interpreted cautiously.

Longitudinal and Control Sample

For a comparison of our longitudinal sample with a control sample, we computed an analysis of variance with the treatment 'sample' as factor.

Results of the Analyses of Variance

Due to some missing data especially in the SES and health ratings, the analyses of variance are based on 93 persons (50 men and 43 women; 23 persons with low SES, 55 with middle and 15 with high SES). The means are weighted according to the cell frequencies.

Time

The scales R_1, R_2, and D_5 yielded significant results. Mean scores on these scales at the four times of measurement are shown in table IV.

In contrast to the findings of *Riegel et al.* (1967), scores decreased over the total longitudinal interval on scales formulated in generalized terms (R_1, D_5) and increased on personal rigidity (R_2), with items stated in the first-person form. The lowest scores were obtained mostly from the second session. Figure 1 illustrates the significant interaction between sex and time on the R_2 scale. Whereas women generally scored lower than men in R_2, they scored higher at measurement point IV.

Table IV. Mean scores on R_1, R_2, and D_5 at all times of measurement for the BLSA

	Measurement point			
	1965/66	1967/68	1969/70	1972/73
R_1	17.8	16.4	17.0	17.4
R_2	14.3	13.8	14.8	15.8
D_5	17.4	16.1	15.9	16.3

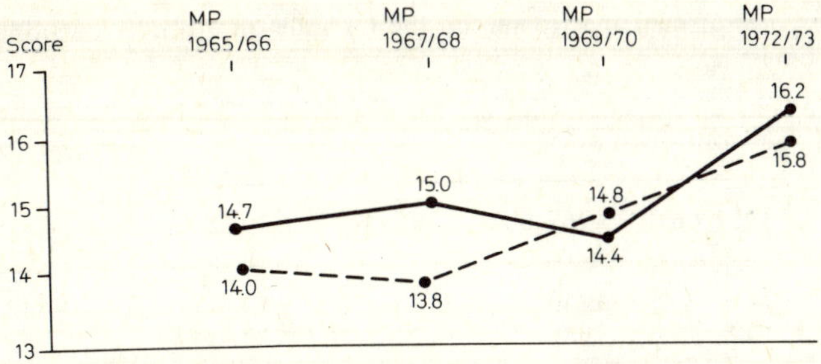

Fig. 1. Mean scores on 'personal rigidity' (R_2) between men (–) and women (– – –) at four measurement points (MP).

Table V. Mean scores of the SES groups on R_1 at all four measurement points

SES	Measurement point				Overall
	1965/66	1967/68	1969/70	1972/73	
Lower	19.4	17.8	18.2	19.8	18.8
Middle	18.3	17.5	17.8	18.2	18.0
Upper	15.9	13.9	15.0	14.1	14.7

Table VI. Mean scores of the SES groups on R_2 at all four measurement points

SES	Measurement point				Overall
	1965/66	1967/68	1969/70	1972/73	
Lower	16.6	15.6	17.1	17.7	16.8
Middle	14.8	14.4	14.7	15.6	14.9
Upper	11.6	11.4	12.6	14.1	12.4

Socioeconomic Status

A significant effect was found for the scales R_1 and R_2. Mean scores on general (R_1) and personal rigidity (R_2) at all measurement points are presented in tables V and VI.

Persons who are classified as lower SES endorse the R_1 items, all of which are expressed in generalized phrases, much more often than persons rated as belonging to middle and upper groups. The results suggest that those subjects

Table VII. Mean scores of men and women on the L_7 scale on attitude toward life at all measurement times

	Measurement point				Overall
	1965/66	1967/68	1969/70	1972/73	
Men	14.9	14.9	14.8	14.8	14.8
Women	13.5	13.0	12.9	12.9	13.1

classified as having lower socioeconomic status also express agreement with personally phrased stereotypes more readily than their counterparts classified as middle and upper SES.

Sex

The L_7 attitude toward life scale produced a significant effect which is illustrated by the means in table VII. Men produced higher scores than women, which indicates that they had a more positive orientation toward life.

Results of Analyses of Covariance

Verbal Intelligence

With verbal intelligence as a covariate, no significant effects ($p < 0.1$) were observed on the R_1 and R_2 scales, where SES was a significant effect with uncontrolled verbal intelligence. There are contrary trends between the sexes in their attitude toward life (L_6) which become more pronounced when verbal intelligence is controlled. Whereas men, who are more negative in their views at the first measurement point, increase in their scores, which means a more and more positive orientation, women, initially more positive in their evaluations, show a decrease in their scores, and this can be interpreted as a more and more negative evaluation of the past and future over the four measurement points. The other reported effects could all be reproduced if verbal intelligence was controlled.

Physician's Health Rating

Ratings by physicians of the subjects' health status reflected longitudinal changes. Observed changes in Riegel scores could be artifacts due to the uncontrolled variable of physical well-being. To rule out this possibility, the analyses of variance were repeated. Taking health data for some subjects caused the

Table VIII. Mean scores on Riegel scales and their standard deviations for samples BLSA (Bonn Longitudinal; n = 119), C (control; n = 57), A_1 (70-year olds, from *Angleitner*, 1972; n = 137), and A_2 (80-year olds, from *Angleitner,* 1972; n = 156)

	BLSA		C		A_1		A_2	
	mean	SD	mean	SD	mean	SD	mean	SD
R_1	17.8	4.8	18.6	3.5	14.4	4.8	16.4	4.5
R_2	15.9	4.4	16.3	5.0	10.4	5.1	12.0	5.2
D_4	4.7	3.5	4.5	2.5	3.2	2.5	3.5	2.4
D_5	16.3	3.5	17.0	4.3	14.6	3.9	16.6	3.8
L_6	14.9	4.5	15.5	5.2	14.4	5.1	12.0	5.0
L_7	14.1	3.3	14.0	4.0	13.3	3.9	13.4	3.3

sample to shrink to 87 persons. Thus, the sample size reduction itself may have influenced the results. All observed effects were replicated. However, the regression coeffients for the health status bound some of the person variance for the scales R_2^{ss}, D_5^{ss}, and L_7^{s}.

Comparison of the Longitudinal and Control Samples

The control sample and the longitudinal sample did not differ significantly from each other in regard to their scores on the Riegel scales at the last time of measurement. A further comparison is offered in table VIII, where data from the longitudinal and control samples are presented with data from the *Angleitner* (1972) sample consisting largely of subjects with higher socioeconomic status. Differences between the present control and longitudinal samples, on the one hand, and the *Angleitner* (1972) samples, on the other hand, follow the lines postulated by *Erlemeier and Angleitner* (1971). The samples with a higher SES rating (A_1 and A_2) express less rigid, intolerant, and dogmatic attitudes, while also holding more negative attitudes toward life than the longitudinal and the control sample.

Discussion

(a) Previous investigations reported little evidence for longitudinal changes over three measurement times from 1965/66 to 1969/70, since longitudinal changes could only account for about 1% of the total variance. The results of the present study lead to the same conclusions for an extended interval of time with four measurement times ranging from 1965/66 to 1972/73. The scales R_1, R_2, and D_5 yield a replicable time effect, but it accounts for only 1–2% of the total variance. Statistically confirmed though it may be, this effect seems inconsequential in terms of the total variance. The other factors account for 1–10% of the total variance, by no means a very promising result.

It can be pointed out that the scores on the scales which are stated in generalized phrases (R_1, D_5) generally decrease, with their lowest points at the second and third measurement points and reflect a slight increase at the fourth measurement point. However, this increase did not reach the level of the first measurement point. But the fact that a new experimenter team administered the test at the fourth measurement point still raises questions as to how the trends in the Riegel scales are best interpreted, in terms of rigidity, etc., or in terms of the changed testing situation.

An increase in rigidity and dogmatism scores with advancing age, such as that reported for the R_1 and D_5 scales by *Riegel and Riegel* (1960) and *Erlemeier and Angleitner* (1971), could not be found for the 7-year period of longitudinal testing. In fact, the significant time effect probably has more to do with a decrease in rigidity scores especially from those testing sessions conducted under equivalent conditions.

However, there was an increase for this time period in 'personal rigidity' (R_2), which suggests that items stated in the first person and relating to concrete situations (by asking what actions the subject would take personally) are more endorsed over our 7-year period. The L_7 scale failed to produce a significant time effect, a finding which is also incongruent with the results of *Riegel et al.* (1967).

All time effects remained significant when the variables 'verbal intelligence' and 'health' were controlled. This indicates that these reported effects are not produced by changes in verbal intelligence or health. The importance of these variables was pointed out by *Angleitner* (1972, 1974b) from findings in his cross-sectional study and it seems that they only apply for cross-sectional samples, but not for a longitudinal sample, which could show more and more selection with the number of measurement points. To prove the latter point we computed the means of our three retested groups in the Riegel scales which they got at the first measurement point. The results are shown in table IX.

It can be said that our sample is not as biased as the results of *Riegel et al.* (1967) would suggest. There is almost no decline over the various retested groups in our attitude scales which would allow us to view our BLSA sample as a 'biased sample' with regard to the Riegel measures. It must be concluded that the postulated claims of controlling the intelligence and health variables regarding rigidity, dogmatism and attitude toward life scales are not as important as was hypothesized from findings of cross-sectional studies.

Table IX. Means at the first testing of the original sample (n = 211) and the retested groups (n = 176 at the second measurement point, n = 143 at the third measurement point, n = 115 at the fourth measurement point) on the Riegel scales

	First measurement point			
	n = 211	n = 176	n = 143	n = 115 (BLSA)
R_1	18.3	18.1	18.2	17.9
R_2	15.2	15.3	15.2	14.7
D_4	4.8	4.8	4.9	4.9
D_5	14.3	14.4	14.5	14.7
L_6	14.3	14.4	14.5	14.7
L_7	14.1	14.5	14.3	14.4

(b) Only few results obtained by cross-sectional comparisons (*Angleitner,* 1972; *Erlemeier and Angleitner,* 1971; *Riegel and Riegel,* 1960; *Riegel et al.*, 1967) could be replicated in this longitudinal study. Longitudinal results remained significant when the variables 'verbal intelligence' and 'health' were controlled as did the above mentioned time effects in the scales R_1, R_2, and D_5, the interaction between sex and time in the R_2 scale, and the sex effect in the attitude toward life scale (L_7). When it came to agreeing with statements phrased in the first-person singular concerning personal reluctance to engage in new activities, as is the case with R_2 items, the financially better-off subjects in our sample showed less reluctant than subjects with lower socioeconomic status. The same is true also for the items of R_1, which are more generally stated. The higher the SES, the lower was the acceptance of the stereotyped phrases. But when verbal intelligence was controlled, this finding could not be replicated. This indicates that the endorsement of stereotyped phrases, regardless of whether they are stated in 'I' or a more general form, is moderated by verbal intelligence, which is generally assumed to be positively correlated with SES.

(c) The finding by *Erlemeier and Angleitner* (1971) that men generally showed a more positive evaluation of their view of present life than women, as reflected in scale items, was also substantiated in this analysis.

Summary

Longitudinal data on an attitude questionnaire by *Riegel and Riegel* (1960) from four times of measurement, 1965/66, 1967/68, 1969/70, and 1972/73, were obtained from 119 subjects. Analyses of variance with the factors sex (masculine/feminine), socioeconomic status (upper/middle/lower), and time (I, II, III, IV) yielded significant time effects for both rigidity scales R_1 and R_2, and the dogmatism scale D_5, significant interactions between sex and time on the R_2 scale, and a significant effect for sex on the L_7 attitude toward life scale. Control of the variable 'verbal intelligence' represented by summed scores on WAIS verbal subtests eliminated the socioeconomic status effect on the R_1 'general rigidity' and R_2 'personal rigidity' scales found in premilinary analyses. A comparison of the longitudinal sample with a similarly recruited and comparable control sample showed no differences in respect to the data of *Riegel and Riegel* (1960).

Contr. hum. Dev., vol. 3, pp. 81–92 (Karger, Basel 1976)

VII. Ecological Correlates of Adjustment to Aging

Ursula Lehr and *Erhard Olbrich*

For about 15 years, ecological factors have received increasing attention as possible determinants of human aging (*Barker and Barker,* 1961; *Radke-Yarrow,* 1963; *Bruhn,* 1971; *Lehr,* 1973). It could be proved empirically that they as well as biosomatic and sociocultural factors (*Thomae,* 1968 a–d; *Havighurst,* 1972) influence the behavior of aged people, above all in the sense of a restriction, a narrowing of their life space, and increasing passivity.

The studies we are referring to analyzed variables like forms of housing and residence, and physical variables. Most important of all were the problems of transportation, and situational factors impairing or facilitating locomotion, like high steps in buses, railway coaches, and escalators. Finally, variables describing accessability of shopping centers and cultural centers were included (*Bruhn,* 1971; *Lehr,* 1973).

Ecological studies done up to now were primarily on macroenvironmental conditions, like life in cities versus life in the country, or regional and cultural differences, etc. rather than on microenvironmental ones. As *Schaie and Gribbin* (1975), we tend to attach importance to the latter, assuming that they are more relevant to an older person's development.

Above all, emphasis on interventional gerontology (*Baltes,* 1973) has directed our attention to ecological variables, especially to those central in an individual's life space (*Lewin,* 1939). One should not underestimate the value of a variety of environmental conditions (e. g. extended green pedestrian signals) for stimulation and activation. Their effect upon an older person's behavior as well as upon his perception of self is remarkable. There are impressive results in intervention gerontology, showing that many forms of enrichment of the environment can successfully stimulate, maintain, and advance psychological processes helpful to the elderly.

Contributions of the Bonn Longitudinal Study on Aging

Within the Bonn Longitudinal Study on Aging (BLSA), underway since 1965 (*Thomae et al.*, 1973), 222 men and women in their sixties and seventies were studied for nearly a decade. Among physical, demographic, social, and psychological variables, some data on the ecological situation of this sample were collected. This definitely offers a chance for a 'study of man, of his total interaction with the universe' (*Lawton and Rich,* 1968). We have attempted to use this very broad definition of ecology, narrowing our approach, however, by selecting specific kinds of ecological variables, and asking the following, more precise, questions.

(1) What is the ecological situation of elderly people who could be followed for 5 years, and how much does it differ for various groups, characterized by differences in sex, age, socioeconomic status (SES), and intelligence? Are there any relevant trends to be detected in the longitudinal observation?

(2) What are the relations between ecological variables and older people's behavior and its cognitive representation?

(3) Finally, the question is raised if there are any functional relations between changes in some ecological variables and the total biographical situation of the aged as it was assessed in 1965, at the beginning of the study.

We had to restrict the set of data considered in this paper to about 100 variables out of the approximately 1,200 that were collected during each of the successive follow-ups of the BLSA. 22 of these were ecological variables in the broad sense of *Lawton et al.* (1968). Descriptive statistics of these were computed, and differences between subgroups were tested. Correlations between ecological variables and biosomatic, psychological, and social characteristics were also computed. Finally, analyses of variance were calculated to check differences between the characteristics of groups showing specific forms of ecological change.

In this study only a 5-year interval (measurement points, MPs, I, III, and IV of the BLSA) is regarded Moreover, the sample was restricted to those 144 older people who had participated in all of the successive follow-ups of the study. They belonged to two cohorts, about 10 years apart in age, one born between 1890 und 1895, the other between 1900 and 1905.

Results

An inspection of our variables roughly following *Thomae's* (1974a) classification of the different meanings of the term ecology, led us to categorize our ecological data as follows:

(1) We could analyze some ecological variables which are descriptive of the *physical environment* of elderly, e. g. the size of the city they live in, the loca-

tion of the apartment (centrally or peripherally in the city), the number of rooms in the apartment, availability of a garden, and ownership status.

(2) We have some variables characterizing the *social environment* of older people: the number of people living in the household, and their relationship to our subjects, and religion, which might indicate a certain type of social environment.

(3) The third group of variables, those which allow an *individual to mold his personal life space,* are income, accessability of a telephone, a car, or the daily newspaper. In this class of variables, we have two relating to expansion of life space in a more literal sense: a rating of the extent of travel, and an index of mobility, i.e. the number of years lived in the same place.

(4) Finally, we have an index of the subject's *cognitive representation of his environment:* a rating of stress experienced from the physical aspect of his housing situation.

Descriptions of the Ecological Situation

(1) Statistical analyses showed that our younger cohort differed only in two of the 22 ecological variables from the older one: subjects in their seventies had lived longer in the same place, and their apartments usually were smaller than those of subjects in their sixties. None of the remaining variables showed any differences between age groups. Developmental changes in such cross-sectional comparisons indicate a rather obvious stability of ecological conditions in the later years of life. We have to be aware, however, that such a generalization can be made only as long as it refers to groups. The comparisons do not fully take account of interindividual differences in measures. These make up a pool of unspecified variance which serves as an error effect in such cross-sectional tests of difference. Although (*Rudinger,* 1971a–c; *Campbell and Stanley,* 1963) repeated measures of the same individuals and ipsative comparisons can show development changes as they occur, they are also liable to error. We will report some results of longitudinal change in a later section of this paper.

(2) As far as stress resulting from one's apartment is concerned, men used to experience it less than women. This was observed throughout the 5-year period under consideration here. According to this sample of variables, men seem to be favored with respect to conditions of their environment. Their ecological situation obviously offers them chances for an extension of various forms of behavior. The question remains to be answered, however, whether men use this chance: in other words, if actual differences in their behavior in contrast to women can be observed (table I).

(3) For comparisons of groups differing in SES, we divided our sample into those above and below a scale score closest to the median (2.92 on a five-point scale). It seems worth noting that neither group differed with respect to living in their own homes, in rented apartments, or in studio apartments. They did not

Table I. Ecological conditions in men and women (for further explanation, see text)

Variable	Men (n = 79; mean/median)	Women (n = 65; mean/median)	Significant difference (t, U or χ^2-test)
Number of years at last address	37.4	34.7	no
Number of people living in			
household	2.4	1.6	yes
MP I	2.4	1.6	yes
MPIII	2.2	1.6	yes
MP IV	2.2	1.5	yes
Stress on account of physical aspects of housing			
MP I[1]	2.1	2.9	yes
MP III[1]	2.6	3.6	yes
MP IV[1]	2.1	2.7	yes
Number of rooms	2.8	2.3	yes
Monthly income			
MP I	831.2	582.4	yes
MP III	951.7	596.1	yes
MP IV	1070.6	788.6	yes
Telephone[2]	2.2	2.2	no
Car[2]	2.4	2.6	no
Newspaper[2]	1.4	2.0	yes
Travel experience[3]	5.7	5.9	no
Living alone	n = 6	n = 35	yes
Living with spouse/children	n = 69	n = 18	yes
Ownership of home			
Owned	n = 33	n = 15	yes
Rented	n = 46	n = 50	yes
Location of home			
Peripheral	n = 49	n = 42	no
Central	n = 29	n = 22	no
City size			
Below 50,000	n = 42	n = 15	yes
Above 50,000	n = 37	n = 50	yes
Garden			
No	n = 28	n = 40	yes
Yes	n = 50	n = 25	yes
Religion			
Catholic	n = 39	n = 27	no
Protestant	n = 31	n = 34	no

1 Scale from 1 = extremely low to 9 = extremely high.
2 Scale from 1 = easily available to 3 = not available.
3 Scale from 1 = little to 9 = much experience.

indicate different degrees of stress resulting from their living situation; location, and situation of their homes seemed comparable (cf. 'garden'). Both groups had a car available to them. It became evident, however, that those in the higher SES had more rooms to live in, and usually shared them with more people. They had more money at their disposal every month, they had a telephone more often, got the daily newspaper more regularly, had travelled more than those of lower SES, and they continued to do so.

What we learn from these differences is that people with a higher SES have a more favorable environment in some psychologically important areas which allows them to expand their social and personal life space. This seems to be a challenge for them, at the same time, to actively engage in broader areas of their life situation. This challenge is accepted in the sense of a chance to avoid restrictions more often imposed on older people of lower SES.

(4) Comparing, finally, those groups made up of people with Wechsler intelligence coefficients below and above a median score, we found significant differences in monthly income. Those with higher intelligence scores usually lived with more people, only seldom alone, and read the newspaper more frequently. From all these data one could say that intelligence is not a variable which, as markedly as SES, is related to different ecological situations. Cross-sectional comparisons show little distinction between elderly people in their sixties or seventies. Ecological situations of the two sexes, however, are markedly different from one another.

Behavioral Correlates of Ecological Variables

We have computed Kendall's τ-coefficients, to find the relationship between ecological variables and the psychological, medical, and social situation of our subjects.

We do not want to go further into the realtionship between ecology and SES or intelligence. This can be inferred from the preceeding part. It seems more important to deal with personality variables now. Among personality dimensions assessed in a behavior rating, developed and refined in several previous studies (*Thomae,* 1968a–d), activity, mood and security showed the clearer, directedness the less distinct relationship to a person's ecological situation. A summary of these coefficients is given in table II. Because some of the data are not measured on ordinal scales, we could not include all ecological variables in this table.

Regarding ecological variables characteristic of subjects *physical environment,* we find rather few correlations to personality dimensions. Still, we can observe that older people living in central parts of cities are more ready to become involved, and are more positive. This is also true for people who have a garden. In general, they indicate more security.

Table II. Correlations between ecological variables and personality ratings (for further explanations, see text)

	City size	Ownership	Location peripheral-central	Garden	Number of rooms	Number of people in household MP I	Number of people in household MP III	Number of people in household MP IV	Monthly income MP I	Monthly income MP III	Monthly income MP IV	Telephone	Car	Newspaper	Travel experience	Number of years at last address	Stress on account of physical aspects of housing MP I	Stress on account of physical aspects of housing MP III	Stress on account of physical aspects of housing MP IV
Activity						+	+	+	+	+	+	+		+	+		–		
Mood			+	+					+		+	+	+	+	+		–	–	
Readiness for involvement	+		+							+	+	+			+				+
Adaptation									+	+	+	+	+	+	+				
Directedness									+	+	+				+				
Security				+		+	+	+	+	+	+	+		+			–		–

With regard to the individual's *social environment,* we find that people living together with several others in their household tend to be more active and indicate more security in the follow-ups of the study. We might add that the older Protestant group had higher activtiy, more positive feelings about everything, more readiness for involvement and displayed a greater feeling of security than Catholics of the same age.

As one might have expected, ecological variables indicating the scope and quality of the *personal life space* showed the most frequent and clearest relation to personality variables. Those with more money had higher values in all personality dimensions considered here in nearly all follow-ups. A similar trend could be observed when availability of a telephone or access to daily news is considered. These are means for an expansion of life space and relate to a person's activity, mood, adaptation, and security. Interestingly enough, availability of a car – a means of locomotion – does not show all these relations. While 'number of years at last address', one index of mobility, shows no relation to any of the personality dimensions, a person's experience and frequency in travelling are positively correlated to nearly all.

In the analysis of *cognitive representations* of one aspect of our subjects' ecological situation, we find that those who feel less stress from problems in the physical situation of the household tend to be more active (at MP I), positive (at MPs I and III), secure (at MPs I and IV), but are less ready to become involved. These results point to the very tentative hypothesis that people with higher ratings in the personality variables considered here tend to have (or have created for themselves) a favorable ecological situation, make better use of it, and are able to master their ecological situation better than those with lower ratings.

In this context, we feel that it is interesting to describe the ecological situation of our sample using two further dimensions: appraisal of the present situation and future plans. Appraisal of the present situation includes the variables (a) satisfaction with present life situation and (b) the feeling of being needed. Those two variables could be summed up to express the extent of successful aging. Future plans include the variables (a) extent of future plans and (b) attitude toward the future.

Older people who live in the center of the city, in smaller towns, without a garden, in larger apartments, or live with others, seem to be more satisfied with their present life situation. They usually have a telephone and a daily newspaper, have lived at the same address longer, travelled more than those who showed less satisfaction, and, in the first year of our study, earned more money.

Close parallels to these relationships can be detected when correlations between a person's sense of being needed and his ecological situation are computed. We found that the feeling of being needed correlates with larger apartment, more people in the household, higher income, availability of telephone, car and newspaper, and more stress on account of the physical aspects of housing, but only at the beginning of the study.

Analyzing the ecological situation of people whose outlook toward the future varies, we find that those who have many plans for 1 year ahead usually live in a larger, rented flat, or have a garden more often. At MP I, we find a significant relationship to larger family living groups. This relationship becomes less significant in the following years. Throughout the period analyzed they have a higher income; newspaper and care are available to them. It is surprising that they have less experience with travelling than those having fewer plans for the future. It might be interesting to find out if this indicates that people accustomed to travel have to restrict their activities, and, parallel to that, their plans, while those who used to be engaged in their closer environment go on to plan more of their activities in this part of their close surroundings.

In former studies we found that one can roughly distinguish between roles in fields closer to the individual and roles in fields more peripheral to him (chap. IX, p. 117; *Munnichs,* 1975). We could show that patterns of longitudinal change indicate a rather high and consistent activity in those more central fields, while less activity is noted in those fields of the social life space considered more peripheral. These and further results indicate a perseverance of higher social competence in areas closer to the aging individual. Now, how does this relate to ecological data?

As summarized in table III we found that subjects living together with more people in their household are more active in their intrafamilial roles (parent, grandparent, spouse) during the first year of the BLSA. This situation becomes less significant in later years. They are, however, more satisfied with these role activities throughout the years we followed them. Such relations between role activities and one index of social environment were reversed for most of the peripheral social roles, especially for the friend, acquaintance, and neighbor roles. Correlations between satisfaction scores and number of people living in one's closest environment were few.

Looking at ecological variables descriptive of what we call the environment's physical properties, we found those older people who lived in smaller cities to be more active in their intrafamilial roles. This could be observed for the kin role as well. People living in larger cities were in general more active in their roles as friend, club member, and citizen. Subjects who had built or purchased their own home were more active as parents, grandparents, and kin. Similarly, taking care of a garden could be observed to go along with high activity as a parent or grandparent. Those living in central parts of cities used to show more activity related to acquaintances; people living in larger flats were more active in their roles as spouse.

Analyzing travelling experiences, we found significant positive covariation with activities as friend and club member, while activities as parent and acquaintance were negatively correlated with this variable. The number of years spent in one place covaried with his activity as a kin and as a club member. People having better chances to form their life space tended to engage more actively in the various forms of social interaction. We are aware that relations found between income and stress arising from the housing situation do not fit into our line of hypothesizing. This may be due to the very rough division we made between role fields. Since their structure is more complicated, we cannot expect distinctions to show up in all single role parameters. This may be complicated even further by our ecological indices differing in their psychological significance for behavior and satisfaction in single roles. Some of these conclusions may not seem to rest on very firm footing, but we believe them to be valuable points to consider for further research. We would, at this point, like to add a thought concerning parallels in correlations between ecological variables and measures of role activity and of satisfaction. Such parallels seem to prevail for the intrafamilial roles. They indicate a congruence in variation of behavioral indices and cognitive representations of behavior. An older person's environment seems to have systematic relation to his overt or manifest action and to awareness of his own activities as well.

Table III. Correlations between ecological variables and social role performance (for further explanation, see text)

	City size	Ownership	Location peripheral-central	Garden	Number of rooms	Number of people in household			Monthly income			Telephone	Car	Newspaper	Travel experience	Number of years at last address	Stress on account of physical aspects of housing		
						MP I	MP III	MP IV	MP I	MP III	MP IV						MP I	MP III	MP IV
Parent																			
Activity	–	–		+		+						+		–			+	–	+
Satisfaction	–		+			+	+	+		–	+	+					+	–	+
Grandparent																			
Activity	–	–		+		+							+				+		+
Satisfaction	–	–		+		+	+	+		–	+						+	–	
Spouse																			
Activity	–				+	+	–		+	+		+	+	+					
Satisfaction				+		+	+	+				+	+	+			+	–	
Kin																			
Activity	–	–							+		+		+		+			+	
Satisfaction	+	–	+	+						–	+			+					
Friend																			
Activity	+					–	–						+		+				
Satisfaction										+		–						–	
Acquaintance																			
Activity				–	–	–	–						+		–				–
Satisfaction	–							+											+
Neighbor																			
Activity					–	–	–		–				+						
Satisfaction	+				–										+		+	–	+
Club member																			
Activity	+					–			+						+	+			
Satisfaction	+									+						+			+
Citizen																			
Activity	+						+			+			+						
Satisfaction								+		+	+			+				–	+

Longitudinal Aspects of Ecological Change

In the following section we will try to analyze to what extent change in three of the ecological variables became evident longitudinally, and how this was influenced by psychological, social, biosomatic, and other ecological variables.

(1) For the whole sample, average monthly income increased between MP I and MP IV. Looking at differences in income of single individuals, however, we found that only 91 had gained (over DM 100.–) more per month after 5 years; 18 of our subjects had lost (more than DM 50.–), and 29 still got about the same income. We checked if these three groups had differed at the beginning of the BLSA. For that purpose we read psychological, social, some medical, and the remaining ecological variables of the subjects belonging to these change groups into the cells of single-factor three-step analysis of variance designs, and tested differences between them. Summarizing variables which differed in these change groups, we tried to identify patterns in older people's situation favoring change over time.

We found 15% of the variables tested this way to differ significantly between groups increasing, descreasing, or not changing in their income. They turned out to be ecological variables mostly: number of people living with our subjects, especially number of single daughters, size of apartment, ownership of home, availability of a car, and daily newspaper. Data on pulmonary volume, number of waking hours per day, lack of impairment in locomotion, and frequency of visits to a restaurant seemed to indicate a person's chance for active participation in everyday life. While these were describing differences observable in manifest behavior, directedness, sense of being needed, and attitudes toward others where regarded to make up inferred personal characteristics influential on the three forms of change.

SES, age, and sex, finally seemed to be indices descriptive of the societal aspects relevant for increase or decrease of income within our society.

(2) Analyzing group changes with respect to number of people living in their household, we found that change of this kind may have been programmed in our subjects life situation in 1965. Most of the significant relationships (18%) were directly describing our subjects' social situation: the number of unmarried children, the number of grandchildren living in the household, and our subjects' activity as parents and acquintance. Others were ecological variables: availability of a telephone, newspaper, and garden. Size of the apartment was different, too. Among the demographic data, age, sex, marital status, and education seemed to influence future change in the size of the group sharing one's household. In addition we found another group of variables to be important: measures of nonverbal intelligence, of psychomotor speed, and of congruence reached between occupational aspirations and achievements. They seem to suggest the scope of achievement an individual can attain.

(3) Regarding differences in degree of stress experienced from physical aspects of the housing situation, we found that change in this variable was related to the following measures of the ecological situation at the beginning of the BLSA, number of grandchildren living in the household, availability of a garden, and getting a pension. Interestingly enough, some indices of an older person's awareness of his social situation could be found to influence development measured in this variable. These were the congruence between what had been expected from members of the family and what these had accomplished, the subject's general attitude toward others, and religious faith. Marital status and age were further variables related to the change. Together with activities of acquaintance and neighbor, and satisfaction with the role, these variables are regarded to be descriptive of social behavior.

A last group of variables needs to be mentioned, characterizing intellectual abilities, and congruence of occupational aspirations and realizations. They, too, were influential in changing stress due to physical aspects of housing.

Discussion

Proceeding in the analysis of our data we sometimes felt our work to be similar to a fishing expedition, throwing nets into unknown waters, and hoping to catch meaningful evidence. Although aware that our results are far from complete, we are confident that we have gained some knowledge in this new field of research: *The* ecology of older people does not exist. Rather it differs from group to group, each of which is characterized by one single or by a pattern of psychological, sociocultural, or physical properties. Trying to identify these appears to be a more fruitful endeavor than cross-sectionally comparing various age groups.

Although all we did in our correlational studies was to search for one-to-one relationships between environmental data and single parameters of older people's total life space, we are impressed by the variety of connexions found. Primarily, relations to variables characterizing behaviorally relevant aspects of the environment and some of the narrower psychological variables proved to be important in these analyses. Congruent interrelations between environment, behavior adjusted to environmental conditions, and cognitive representation of this behavior are most impressive. So, type und intensity of environmental stimulation appear to be important factors for development in old age. In this process the individual by no means is a mere passive recipient of stimulation. Adaptation and creation of congruence seem to be two-way processes going on between the elderly and their environment (*Schooler,* 1969; *Brown,* 1965).

This view is supported by our longitudinal analysis of a small segment of this process. Following our subjects over time suggested that ecological change depends upon, or is programmed by, rather complex life situations which best can be described as pattern of ecological, psychological, social and medical factors. We will elaborate on these configurations, before all trying to identify the psychological process that appears while change in later life occurs.

Contr. hum. Dev., vol. 3, pp. 93–112 (Karger, Basel 1976)

VIII. Perceived Life Space: Patterns of Consistency and Change

Hermann-Josef Fisseni

Introduction

Concepts, Theory, Background

The concept of 'life space', introduced by *Lewin* (1963), comprehends all that is 'real to a subject', thus not meaning objective reality in itself, but 'things' as seen, felt, evaluated by a person. In terms of 'cognitive theory of behavior' (*Baldwin,* 1969, p. 326) the concept of life space can be defined as 'the cognitive representation of the distal environment' that 'acts as the effective environment which . . . guides overt behavior toward its target or goal'. The dynamic aspect of this concept is stressed by *Bottenberg* (1970, p. 415) who, following *Leeper* (1965), states that 'processes of perception which represent cognition in a broader sense contain as an essential part a motivating variable that arouses, keeps working and directs behavior'. The dynamic components of the concept of life space will be used to explain the results gained in this study.

It is intended to use data of the Bonn Longitudinal Study of Aging (BLSA; chap. I, p. 1) for examining the process of aging by analyzing some dimensions of life space, assuming that change or consistency in this cognitive representation of the environment is related to changes in motivation and emotion and to changes in overt behavior.

Under the same aspect, a portion of the data to be used in this study was analyzed by *Opgenoorth* (1971). To describe the life space of 187 participants of the BLSA at its third measurement point (MP) in 1967, he introduced 25 variables reflecting individual views of environment. The most influential variables for this subjective outlook proved to be state of health, attitude toward present and future life situation, structure of personality (as measured by behavior ratings) and, most important, intelligence. *Opgenoorth* (1971) found that the subjects tried to bring their conceptual and motivational systems into congruence – especially by adapting the cognitive system (e. g. judgments about past life, conclusions for present and future situations) to emotional needs; and that in persons who were judged to age successfully the different sections of life space proved to be in a high degree of concordance.

Method

Examining change and consistency in life space over a period of years can be undertaken in two ways: (a) by considering individuals who are identical in respect to certain characteristics of life space, and comparing divergence or convergence of their behavior; (b) by tracing identical traits and their constellation in life space, and verifying whether regular configurations turn up due to age, sex, health, and other variables influencing the process of aging. The first approach will be reserved for a broader study of the BLSA data. The second is followed in this paper. Both these methods can be used as instruments of differential psychology insofar as typical behavior patterns are investigated.

The statistical method to be used will be the 'configural frequency analysis' (CFA), developed by *Lienert and Krauth* (1975). This method allows a decision as to whether the frequencies with which some constellations of variables turn up are significant enough to characterize a group of individuals. In this sense it is also a method of differential psychology. An advantage of this instrument is that it makes both longitudinal and cross-sectional consideration possible. A disadvantage is the fact that in our sample it is applicable to relatively small sets of variables.

Sample

The sample to be analyzed is that of the BLSA (for details, see chap. III, p. xxx). Subjects of the study were seen repeatedly at approximately 2-year intervals. Data from all of the five MPs were included in this study. For longitudinal considerations, only the data of the 121 survivors were analyzed. For cross-sectional evaluations, the sample of nonsurvivors is also included, but this will be mentioned explicitly in each case.

Aspects of Life Space

Three aspects of life space will be studied: (1) an example for the extent of life space will be given by considering some significant objects that stand out in subjective environment; (2) another group of statements is related to the perception of stress or conflict, and (3) a further set of data is used to evaluate the quality of life space by gathering information about subjective life satisfaction. It must be admitted that this selection proves a far from complete analysis of individual life space. It can only be considered an example of its different dimensions.

The information was drawn from three interviews per MP covering present, past, and future situations of the subjects. Rating scales (from 1 to 9) were used for measuring these aspects. For statistical purposes, these ratings were transformed into scores 'above' or 'below' the grand median, i. e. the median over five MPs.

Results

The results of each set of ratings will be presented separately. First, the statistical values will be presented (a figure showing the longitudinal distribution of medians; scores of intercorrelations and of reliability). Second, the findings on change and consistency of life space dimensions will be summarized. Change means that a pattern of behavior, considered longitudinally, is different at different MPs (the statistical significance being measured by the CFA). In an analogous way, consistency means that a pattern of behavior is, considered statistically, the same at different MPs. Consistency and change – it may be repeated – is referred to only with respect to the group of 121 survivors (for the problems that arise from the longitudinal measurements of change, see chap. III, p. 12; a short discussion is given also in this chapter, p. 95). Third, the influence of external variables will be tested (e. g. age, sex, health, socioeconomic status – SES).

Change and Consistency in the Extension of Life Space

To represent the extension of life space, three ratings have been selected as significant objects standing out in the subjective environment. These ratings cover attitude towards other people, anticipation of future life situation, and extent of making plans. Data have been collected at MPs I, III and IV.

Reliablility was measured as 'test' at MP I and 'retest' at MPs III and IV. The scores are as follows: $r_{others} = 0.75$, $r_{plans} = 0.43$, $r_{future} = 0.67$. Here we are already faced with the question of change and consistency. The scores indicate some change over the different MPs. Otherwise the coefficients should be higher. Yet, where is the change to be sought, in the dimension measured or in the instrument measuring the dimension? Is life space changing (the instrument being consistent)? Is the instrument changing (life space remaining consistent)? Or is change resulting from both these influences? (For a full discussion of this problem, see chap. III, p. 12.) The difficulty of answering these questions must be kept in mind, when interpreting our findings; every interpretation must be very cautious.

The intercorrelations between the three ratings (given as the mean of Spearman's ρ) vary from MP to MP. (MP I: $\rho = 0.46$; MP III: $\rho = 0.23$; MP IV: $\rho = 0.21$; grand mean over all MPs: $\rho = 0.35$). This result seems to stress the fact that the three dimensions change relatively independently from each other. Otherwise the coefficients should be nearly the same at each MP. This change might be illustrated by figure 1, showing the medians at the three MPs. Our major interest was to find out whether certain patterns in the extension of life space would emerge over all MPs and which differences would turn up between the different MPs.

Evaluating the data over the three MPs, four patterns of changing and consistent behavior are recognizable. Pattern A: a group of old people scoring high in all of the three aspects (others, making plans, future); pattern B: a group scoring high in making plans and looking forward to the future, but scoring low in attitude towards others; pattern C: a group scoring high in attitude towards others, but scoring low in making plans and anticipation of the future; pattern D: a group scoring high in attitude towards others and anticipation of the future, but scoring low in making plans.

The patterns of change and consistency, as expressed in the ratings, can best be seen in table I that delineates whether a group characterized by a pattern is growing stronger from one MP to another (increase), or is becoming smaller (decline), or whether no change at all is occurring (consistency).

Table I indicates that patterns A and B are attenuating from I to III, but remain consistent from III to IV. Patterns C and D go the opposite way. They grow stronger from I to III, but then become steadier from III to IV. Generalizing these results would mean that change takes place from MP I to MP III, and consistency is observed from MP III to MP IV.

This interpretation is supported by a cross-sectional survey that also includes the nonsurvivors of our sample: in MP I two patterns are significant, one characterized by high scores and the other by low scores. The remarkable point, under the aspect of cognitive theory, is the fact that only the two groups who are positively or negatively orientated on all three dimensions contrast with each other, thus favoring the hypothesis that the different systems adapt to one another. In MPs III and IV no significant pattern emerges (although in MPs III a tendency towards the two patterns stated in MP I is recognizable).

Age

Introducing calendar age as a discriminant variable (in a one-way design) brings about a moderate effect: three patterns of change and consistency emerge. Pattern A: a 'younger' group (60–70 years) scores high in all of the three dimensions (others, plan-making, future); pattern B: an 'older' group (70–80 years) gets high scores in plan-making and in anticipation of the future and low scores in attitude towards others; pattern C: an 'older' group gets high scores in attitude towards others and low scores in making plans and in anticipating the future. Table II illustrates the directions of change and the tendencies of consistency again. On the whole, table II indicates that, as in the preceding consideration, change takes place from MP I to MP III, and that consistency can be seen from MP III to MP IV.

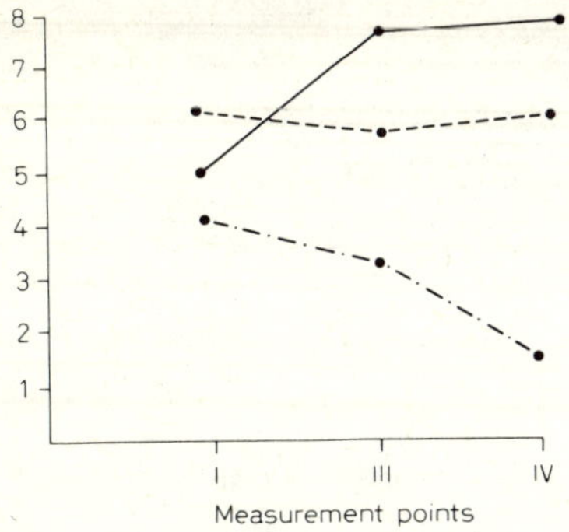

Fig. 1:. Subjective view of characteristic 'objects' in elderly persons' life space (medians over three MPs). – = Others; ––– = future; ·–· = plan-making.

Table I

Pattern	Score		MP	
	high	low	I–III	III–IV
A	others, plans, future	–	decline	consistency
B	plans, future	others	decline	(tendency to increase)
C	others	plans, future	increase	consistency
D	others, future	plans	increase	(tendency to decline)

Table II

Pattern	Score		MP	
	high	low	I–III	III–IV
'Younger' group				
A	others, plans, future	–	(tendency to decline)	consistency
'Older' group				
B	plans, future	others	decline	(tendency to increase)
C	others	plans, future	increase	consistency

Table III

Pattern	Score		MP	
	high	low	I–III	III–IV
Women				
A	others, plans, future	–	decline	(tendency to increase)
Men				
B	plans, future	others	decline	consistency
C	others, future	plans	increase	decrease

A cross-sectional evaluation including the nonsurvivors is added, supporting the longitudinal results. In MP I two sets of groups turn out to be significant, each set comprehending a 'younger' and an 'older' group. Set A consists of those (younger and older) who have widened life space extension, set B of those (younger and older) for whom it is reduced. This result of older and younger having the same pattern of behavior shows most clearly that it is not calendar age that has decisive bearings on forming life space extension, but that other variables (not tested here) are of greater influence. In MP III only one group proves characteristic, 'older' people having reduced life space dimensions. In MP IV no pattern is found to be significant.

Sex

Discriminating our sample under the aspect of sex difference (again in a one-way design) shows some distinctions. Three patterns can be observed. Pattern A: women scoring high on all three aspects; pattern B: men scoring high in plan-making and anticipation of the future, but low in attitude towards other people; pattern C: men scoring high in attitude towards others and in anticipating the future, but low in making plans. Table III explains change and consistency turning up from MP I to MP IV. In table III more variations of change and consistency are indicated than in the preceding considerations, though the overall impression remains the same. It is especially from MP I to MP III that change is going on. From MP III to MP IV, consistency is 'preserved', except for pattern C which also changes from MP III to MP IV.

A cross-sectional evaluation, including also the nonsurvivors, draws a similar picture. In MP I two groups emerge as characteristic. Group A comprehends a subgroup of males and a subgroup of females, both having reduced dimensions of life space. Group B also consists of a subgroup of males and a subgroup of females, yet both have widened life space dimensions. Here an interpretation is called for that regards the subjective implications of the divergence and convergence among the two sexes. A cognitive theory of behavior can yield such an interpretation as will be explained. In MP III only one group stands out, the men with reduced life space extension. In MP IV no pattern emerges as characteristic.

Table IV

Pattern	Score high	Score low	MP I–III	MP III–IV
Good health				
A	others, plans, future	–	decline	consistency
B	plans, future	others	decline	consistency
Poor health				
C	others	plans, future	consistency	(tendency to increase)

Health

According to different states of health (considered in a one-way design), three different patterns of change and consistency in life space extension can be distinguished. Pattern A: a group of those in good health who score high in all of the three dimensions tested; pattern B: a group of those in good health who score high in plan-making and in anticipation of the future and score low in attitude towards others; pattern C: a group of those in poor health who score high in attitude towards other people and score low in plan-making and anticipation of the future. Table IV illustrates change and consistency. We find essentially the same picture as before: change from MP I to MP III, consistency from MP III to MP IV.

The cross-sectional evaluation, including all nonsurvivors, does not create a different impression. In MP I three patterns turn up: A: a small group characterized by better health, but by reduced life space extension; B: a larger group with significantly better health and widened life space dimensions, and C: a third group in poor health and with a correspondingly reduced life space extension. In MP III only one pattern proves characteristic: poor health in connection with reduced life space. In MP IV no significant group shows up.

Socioeconomic Status

With respect to SES it is interesting that significant patterns turn up only among those with higher SES. Pattern A: high SES, scoring high in all three dimensions; pattern B: high SES, scoring high in plan-making and in anticipating the future, but scoring low in attitude towards others; pattern C: high SES, scoring high in attitude towards others, but scoring low in making plans and in anticipation of the future; pattern D: high SES, scoring high in attitude towards other people and in anticipating the future, but scoring low in making plans. Table V confirms the patterns of change and consistency already established: change from MP I to MP III, consistency from MP III to MP IV.

Table V

Pattern	Score		MP	
	high	low	I–III	III–IV
High SES				
A	others, plans, future	–	decline	consistency
B	plan, future	others	decline	consistency
C	others	plans, future	decline	consistency
D	others, future	plans	decline	consistency

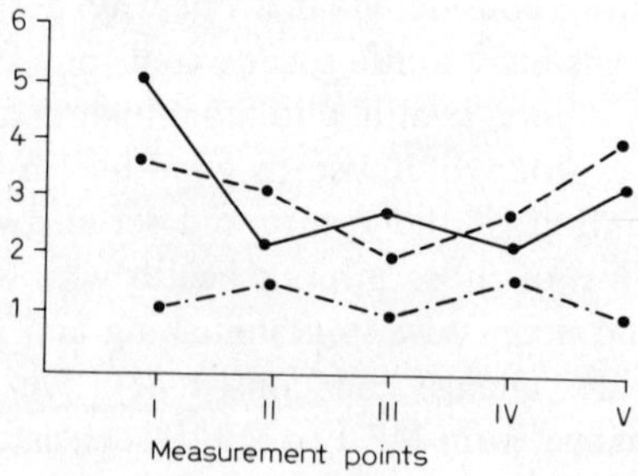

Fig. 2. Stress and/or conflict in dimensions of elderly persons' life space (medians over five MPs). ––– = Health; – = family; ·–· = housing.

Table VI

Pattern	Stress		MP			
	low	high	I–II	II–III	III–IV	IV–V
A	family health, housing	–	decline	increase	increase	decline
B	–	family, health, housing	consistency	decline	decline	increase
C	family	health, housing	consistency	consistency	consistency	increase

Change and Consistency in the Perception of Stress or Conflict

In our evaluation of the BLSA data we decided to use the following variables for the description of perceiving stress or conflict: reported difficulties about family life (spouse, relatives, offspring); worries about health; housing problems. Data are available for all five MPs.

The intercorrelations of the three ratings (Spearman's ρ) show that the fields represented are relatively independent from each other (MP I: $\rho = 0.22$; MP II: $\rho = 0.13$; MP III: $\rho = 0.20$; MP IV: $\rho = 0.20$; MP V: $\rho = 0.25$; grand mean over all measurement points: $\rho = 0.20$). The reliablility scores are more balanced here than above: $r_{housing} = 0.67$; $r_{health} = 0.69$; $r_{family} = 0.61$. This indicates considerable consistency. The longitudinal distribution of the medians is given in figure 2.

In longitudinal examination of the five MPs three patterns show up. Pattern A: a group claiming not to be affected at all by the three themes introduced; pattern B: a group feeling highly stressed by all of three kinds of burdens; pattern C: a group denying housing stress, yet admitting being burdened by questions of health and family life. Under the aspect of a cognitive interpretation it is interesting that the two groups with 'clear-cut' profiles (A: all scores above; B: all scores below the median) show the largest part of change. Here the process of one behavior system being adapted to another can be studied most clearly.

A cross-sectional evalution is added, including also the nonsurvivors. At MP I one pattern turns up, characterizing a group feeling stressed by all of the three aspects tested, the conflict resulting especially from housing questions and family life. In MP II no significant pattern is recognizable. In MP III a pattern appears which is the opposite of that at MP I, namely a group who claims not to feel stressed at all. Here it is the question of housing (equal to MP I) and of health (unequal to MP I) that contribute most to form the 'new' pattern. In MP IV no characteristic pattern emerges. At MP V the same pattern is outstanding as in MP III: a group not worried at all about the three themes under consideration.

Age

Introducing age as an external variable (in a one-way design) has a discriminating effect. There are four patterns emerging that describe significant changes. Pattern A: 'younger' old people (60–70 years), and pattern B: 'older' people (70–80 years) who do not feel stressed; pattern C: 'younger' old people, bothered by housing problems and family life, but not by questions of health; pattern D: 'older' people who feel burdened by all of the three problems mentioned. Table VII illustrates change and consistency over the different MPs, as represented in the ratings. Under the aspect of a cognitive theory it is interesting that the outstanding patterns are those having all scores at the same level, namely all above the median (thus indicating low stress in all dimensions tested). Again, an interpretation is suggested that assumes different dimensions to be adapted to each other.

Table VII

Pattern	Stress low	Stress high	MP I–II	MP II–III	MP III–IV	MP IV–V
'Younger' group						
A	family, health, housing	–	consistency	consistency	increase	consistency
'Older' group						
B	family, health, housing	–	consistency	increase	increase	decline
'Younger' group						
C	health	family, housing	consistency	consistency	decline	consistency
'Older' group						
D	–	family, health, housing	consistency	decline	consistency	increase

The cross-sectional consideration may serve as a supplement, including the non-survivors. Patterns turn up only at MP III, but in a paradoxical sense. A group of 'older' people (70–80 years) emphasizes not feeling burdened at all; a group of 'younger' ones (60–70 years) says that they feel strong conflicts in family, health, and housing problems.

Sex

Distinguishing males and females over the five points of measurement (in a one-way design) shows one clear effect. Pattern A: a group of men is characterized by not complaining at all about any of the possible conflicts considered; pattern B: a group of women is characterized by not complaining at all about any of the possible conflicts considered. Change and consistency within these two groups are shown in table VIII. Change is found to a larger extent in the male group. In the female one there is a greater amount of consistency over the years. But the direction of change in the two groups seems opposite. In the female group a tendency is recognizable towards steadying the pattern of not complaining, whereas among the men on the whole this pattern rather fades away.

Table VIII

Pattern	Stress		MP			
	low	high	I–II	II–III	III–IV	IV–V
Men						
A	family, health, housing	–	decline	increase	consistency	decline
Women						
B	family, health, housing	–	consistency	consistency	increase	consistency

Table IX

Pattern	Stress		MP			
	low	high	I–II	II–III	III–IV	IV–V
Poor health						
A	family, health, housing	–	consistency	consistency	increase	decline
B	family, health	housing	consistency	consistency	increase	decline
Good health						
C	housing	family, health	consistency	consistency	consistency	increase

The cross-sectional evaluation shows a picture of remarkable variation. Here the non-survivors are included. At MPs I and II the significant patterns are similar. A male group denies being stressed. A female group asserts that they feel heavily under stress. It is housing problems and questions of family life that bother women the most. Men do not mention similar difficulties. At MP III a slight change takes place. The two groups turn up again, females suffering stress, males not at all. But it is now family and health (not family and housing) about which old women, but not old men are worried. At MP VI only the male group remains in evidence. In MP V two (small) female groups can be observed, one denying, the other suffering stress in the fields mentioned.

Health

Regarding state of health (again, in a one-way design), change and consistency are observed in three significant patterns. Pattern A: a group of those in poor health, but having no complaints about the three problems considered; pattern B: a group characterized by poor health and by complaints about housing problems, but not worried about family life or state of health; pattern C: a third group described as being in good health, yet feeling worried about state of health and family life, but not housing problems. As table IX illustrates, in the first years consistency can be observed, in the last years it is change that prevails.

The cross-sectional consideration, including the nonsurvivors, draws the following picture. At MPs I and II a group of aged persons in poor health affirm that they feel molested in all of the three fields investigated. At MPs III and IV a pattern turns up characterizing those in a better state of health and, so to speak, with concomitant freedom from stress in the three problem areas mentioned. At MP V no significant pattern emerges.

Socioeconomic Status

As in the preceding paragraph, significant patterns turn up only among those old people with higher socioeconomic status. Three patterns describe change and consistency: (A) a group of high SES persons, emphasizing the absence of stress due to housing problems, family life or state of health; (B) a group of high SES persons, unburdened by housing problems, yet worried about family and health problems; and (C) a group of high SES persons, not bothered about state of health, but concerned about problems of housing and family life. Table X delineates change and consistency over the years. Only in the last years does change come about. During the first years consistency is preserved within the patterns tested.

Table X

Pattern	Stress		MP			
	low	high	I–II	II–III	III–IV	IV–V
High SES						
A	family, health, housing	–	(tendency to decline)	(tendency to increase)	increase	decline
B	housing	family health	consistency	consistency	consistency	increase
C	health	family, housing	consistency	consistency	decline	consistency

Change and Consistency in the Quality of Life Space

For the evaluation of life space quality, three variables were selected as representing satisfaction with present life situation: attitude toward the present, perceived variability of daily life, and feeling needed by others (the addition of the third scale is based on *Opgenoorth,* 1971, pp. 168–169.)

The intercorrelations (Spearman's ρ) remain rather low (MP I: $\rho = 0.25$; MP III: $\rho = 0.30$; MP IV: $\rho = 0.17$; grand mean over all MPs: $\rho = 0.24$). So it might be assumed that the three dimensions represent three relatively independent aspects. The reliability scores are satisfactory: $r_{present} = 0.74$; $r_{variability} = 0.60$; $r_{needed} = 0.75$. Data were collected at MPs I, III and IV. The longitudinal distribution of their medians is shown in figure 3.

A longitudinal consideration proves consistency and change to be given in a significant degree by two patterns. Pattern A: a group of old people, who report that their daily routine varies little and who show a rather negative attitude toward the present, but feel needed by other people in a remarkable measure; pattern B: a group with a negative orientation toward the present, but reporting a good deal of variability in their daily life and who feel needed by other people. The pattern of change and consistency in these patterns is shown in table XI. Table XI indicates that the group characterized by pattern A does not vary markedly from MP I to MP III, but does grow significantly stronger from MP III to MP IV, whereas the group described by pattern B is reduced from MP I to MP III, and then varies only within the limits of statistical confidence from MP III to MP IV.

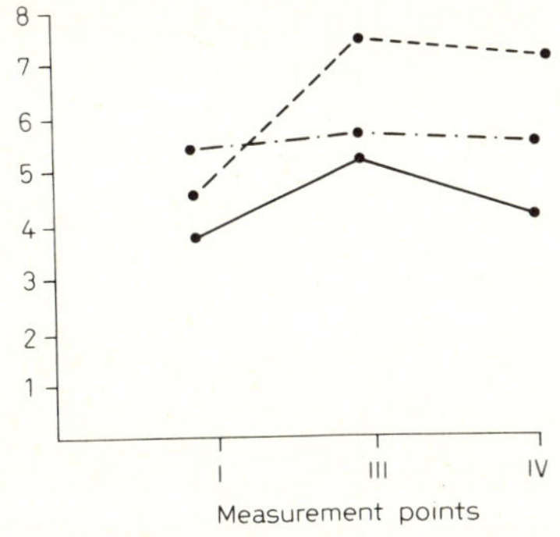

Fig. 3. Perception of present life situation: an example of quality of elderly persons' life space (medians over three MPs). ––– = Present; ·–· = being needed; – = daily life.

Table XI

Pattern	Score: high	Score: low	MP: I–III	MP: III–IV
A	being needed	variability, present	consistency	increase
B	present	variability, being needed	decline	consistency

Table XII

Pattern	Score: high	Score: low	MP: I–III	MP: III–IV
'Older' group				
A	being needed	variability, present	consistency	increase
'Younger' group				
B	variability, being needed, present	–	increase	consistency

Table XIII

Pattern	Score: high	Score: low	MP: I–III	MP: III–IV
Women				
A	being needed	variability, present	consistency	increase
Men				
B	being needed, present	variability	increase	decline
C	variability	being needed, present	(tendency to increase)	decline
D	variability, being needed	present	decline	consistency

A cross-sectional evaluation including the nonsurvivors brings the following results. At MP I, two combinations prevail, one group having scores below, the other one above the median. This means that there exist two patterns of life space quality, one characterized by satisfaction with, the other one by rejection of present life situation. At MP III the two patterns (above and below median) turn up again. At MP IV no pattern appears distinctly. Only a tendency is observable towards forming the group above median (= showing satisfaction with present situation).

Age

Calendar age, as a discriminant variable (introduced in a one-way design), proves effective in 'creating' only two patterns. Pattern A: a group of 'older' people (70–80 years), characterized by high scores in the dimension of feeling needed by others, yet by low scores with respect to variability of daily life and attitude toward the present; pattern B: a 'younger' group (60–70 years), having high scores under all aspects tested. Table XII illustrates change and consistency as expressed in the ratings over the different MPs. As table XII shows, the same pattern as in the preceding consideration turns up again here. Pattern A is the same in both cases, also with regard to consistency and change. Patern B is interesting under the aspect of cognitive interpretation: it might be an example, again, of the different systems (cognitive and emotional) adapting to one another.

A cross-sectional consideration shows different patterns for different MPs. Nonsurvivors are included. At MP I three patterns emerge: A: an 'older' group, characterized by little satisfaction with present life situation (all scores below median); B: an 'older' group, taking the opposite stand, namely that they are satisfied with the actual situation under all aspects considered, and C: a third group of 'younger' old people, having the same scores (all above median) as group B. Especially the contrast between pattern A and B calls for an explanation which pays heed to the subjective components of behavior. Given the same data (age and three variables tested), the outcome is divergent, thus implying a different subjective 'interpretation' (= adaptation) of the behavior systems. At MP III the same patterns emerge as at MP I. At MP IV only pattern C turns up ('younger', satisfied under all aspects considered).

Sex

Comparing our sample under the aspect of sex differences, the following patterns turn up. Pattern A: a group of women, claiming to feel highly needed by others, yet having little variability in daily life and rather negatively oriented to the present; pattern B: a group of old men, scoring high in attitude toward the present and in feeling needed by others and scoring low only in estimated variability of daily life; pattern C and D: groups of old men differing only in scores of 'being needed' by others, as can be seen in table XIII. It is rather surprising that the pattern characterizing the group of women does not occur among the groups of men. In addition, it is interesting to see that there is more change going on than consistency being preserved.

This variety of patterns can also be observed in the cross-sectional comparisons, including the nonsurvivors. At MP I two opposite groups turn up, a completely dissatisfied female one and a male group who are completely satisfied with the present life situation under all aspects tested. At MP III the scene changes. A group of males as well as a group of fermale one and a male group who are completely satisfied with the present life situation under all aspects tested. At MP III the scene changes. A group of males as well as a group of females express their dissatisfaction and a group of males as well as a group of females claim to be highly satisfied with the present situation. At MP IV the multiple patterns continue to appear. Two female groups emerge characterized by opposite tendencies, one by satisfaction, the other one by discontent. Two male groups turn up, both partially content, partially discontent, with satisfaction and dissatisfaction covering different dimensions. On the whole, here again the data lend themselves to an explanation using terms of cognitive theory because, so to speak, the same 'original' data (namely sex and the variables tested) are subjectively expressed in different patterns.

Health

Distinguishing groups (in a one-way design) according to different states of health, three patterns appear. Pattern A: a group of those in a state of good health, scoring high in their judgment of daily variability and feeling needed by others, and scoring low in their attitude towards the present; pattern B: a group of those in poor health, scoring low in their attitude to the present and their judgment about daily life, and scoring high in being needed by others; pattern C: a third group of those in poor health, scoring high in their judgment on variability of daily life, and scoring low in their feelings of being needed by other people and in their attitude towards the present. The patterns of change and consistency are shown in table XIV. The difficulty in interpreting these patterns lies in the fact that no regularity explaining the details is recognizable.

Table XIV

Pattern	Score		MP	
	high	low	I–III	III–IV
Good health				
A	variability, needed	present	decline	consistency
Poor health				
B	being needed	variability, present	consistency	increase
C	variability	being needed, present	increase	consistency

From the cross-sectional consideration, including the nonsurvivors, the following picture can be drawn. At MP I two opposite groups prevail, both creating, so to speak, congruity between state of health and the dimensions tested. One group is characterized by poor health and low scores in the three ratings, the other one by good health and high scores in the three dimensions. At MP III the same patterns emerge, but one more group comes up, significant by having poor health and stating complete satisfaction. Perhaps it is this latter group for which a cognitive concept of interpretation can be justified most easily. At MP IV only one group stands out: those in good health who assert their satisfaction on all aspects tested.

Socioeconomic Status

Using SES as a discriminant variable (in a one-way design), only one pattern characterizing change and consistency longitudinally turns up in our sample: an upper SES group with high scores in attitude towards the present and feeling needed by other people, and low scores in assessments of the variability of daily life. This group grows stronger from MP I to MP III, yet is reduced again from MP III to MP IV.

Summary and Discussion

It was the intention of this study to examine the process of aging by analyzing some dimensions of life space and then to evaluate these dimensions within the frame of reference of a cognitive theory of behavior.

Introducing cognitive concepts to explain the findings is not to say that other theories would not be applicable, but it means that a cognitive interpretation is very (even most) adequate for the data under consideration. The variables studied were not meant to represent objective conditions, e. g., of family life or of housing problems, as described by objective observers. They were conceived of as expressions of subjective attitudes or personal 'comments' on important topics in the aging process. In other words, the information gathered was meant to cover sections of life space, not objects of the 'real' world. So it is but consequent to explain the data by a theory corresponding to this viewpoint.

A difficulty is connected with this interpretation. It is assumed that change and consistency expressed in the ratings reflect change and consistency in behavior (and not primarily in the process of measurement). The problem is that of the reliability (and validity) of our rating scales. This question is discussed by *Rudinger* (chap. III, p. 12); it was mentioned at the beginning of this chapter (p. 95) and is repeated here in order to point to the caution to be used in our interpretations.

In addition to these problems, certain difficulties resulted from the statistical method used here, the CFA. Only a small set of variables could be considered at a time, but these could be tested cross-sectionally as well as longitudinally. But there is no criterion for deciding in advance which variables should be grouped together and analyzed using the CFA. In this study this question was dealt with by checking the intercorrelations between the variables selected. A further disadvantage was the fact that, with respect to our sample, only one-way designs were applicable in introducing external variables (age, sex, health, SES being tested only separately). More efficiency should be expected from multivariate methods. It is planned to introduce such methods in reanalyzing the BLSA data concerning subjective life space. In this study it was intended to give but an example of the varying processes of aging as considered under the aspect of perceived life space dimensions.

Turning to the findings and weighing them as a whole, it might be said that change is observed to a larger extent than consistency. Evaluating such a result in terms of cognitive theory, this would indicate that, in life space of the aged people in this study, characteristics of 'fluid' cognitive compounds predominate over those of 'crystallized' quality, thus expressing the adaptation of cognitive and motivational systems to each other. Yet, the extent of consistency stated in the results reflects the importance of the 'conservative' force to keep the different behavior systems in balance.

Applying this general interpretation to the three dimensions considered, it can be seen that change in life space extension occurs primarily from MP I to MP III, whereas consistency is observed primarily from MP III to MP IV. For perceived stress, the opposite is true. More consistency is observed during the first measurement points than during the last ones. As to life space quality, both consistency and change are coexistent to a larger extent than above. From these observations it follows that the more 'fluid' force (of adapting behavior systems to each other) and the more 'crystallized' force (of keeping them in balance) cannot be attributed to special time spans or special behavior systems, but are embedded in a more complex network of variables. A similar overall result can be summarized regarding the influence of the external variables tested.

To begin with, there is no recognizable regularity in this study which explains the effect of calendar age. There are 'constellations' of variables which could be attributed to the influence of age, e. g. when 'younger' subjects have higher scores in all dimensions tested (life space extension: attitude towards others, plan-making, anticipation of the future, p. 96; life space quality: judgment on the variability of daily life, feeling needed by others, attitude towards the present, p. 106). This constellation seems to correspond with an age-determined pattern ('youth' = widened life space). Yet, the counterpart ('older age' = reduced life space) does not turn up in our longitudinal schemes, and, still more important, the youth-determined pattern tends to diminish from MP I to MP III (p. 96). As to life space quality, the association of old age with reduced life space increases from MP I to MP III. Furthermore, as to perceived stress, a set of constellations turns up which contrast with the results discussed so far.

There are constellations showing the same pattern for 'older' and 'younger' subjects (low stress with respect to family, health, and housing problems, cf. pp. 101–102). This result of 'older' and 'younger' having the same behavior pattern is best explained in cognitive terms. It is not age according to which the variables are being 'put to work', but a model in which other variables serve as centers of 'constellation'. 'Older' people in better health might adapt the different systems to this better state, for example.

This cognitive interpretation is confirmed by evaluating single cross-sectional findings. There are 'older' groups having the same pattern as corresponding 'younger' groups, e. g. in life space extension (p. 98). There are groups of the same age having contrasting behavior patterns, e. g. 'older' people having high scores in all variables tested versus 'older' people having low scores in all variables (cf. life space quality, p. 106). Finally, there are groups characterized by paradoxical constellations, e. g. 'younger' old people admitting suffering under stress, and 'older' people maintaining that they do not (cf. p. 102).

From all these results it follows that the life space dimensions tested in this study are affected only to a small extent by chronological age, as defined by the two cohorts included in our study.

Evaluating the influence of sex differences, it may be stated that more change shows up within the male than within the female group (this effect cannot be attributed to sampling bias, the quotas of males and females, on the whole, being fairly balanced). A reason for this disproportion could not be found in this study.

Some findings call for an interpretation based on the subjective adaption process differentiating males and females. The cognitive concept of 'knowing' one's sex role and adapting one's behavior to this role system offers itself as a rationale for some results, primarily in cross-sectional comparisons. As to perceived stress (p. 103) or life space quality (p. 108), patterns of aging correspond with such an explanation. The women feel stressed, but not the men; the women feel complete dissatisfaction, the men complete satisfaction; the women are worried by womanlike problems (family life and housing problems, cf. p. 103), but the men are not. Such statements fit in with this sex-determined interpretation. Thereby, it may be repeated, it is not assumed that women are stressed, and men are not. It is only supposed that these statements reflect the subjective view of dominant problems in old age and the influence of this view on the whole of behavior.

Yet, there are findings that cannot be explained in this way. Men and women characterized by the same pattern, e. g. male and female groups having reduced or widened space dimensions (as to attitude towards others, plan-making and anticipation of the future, cf. p. 98); male and female groups assuring their complete satisfaction or dissatisfaction with present life situation (cf. p. 108): such results cannot be explained by sex difference, but call for other subjectively prevailing themes (not tested here) which influence behavior according to this predominance.

So, as in the case of calendar age, a cognitive interpretation of findings with respect to sex differences leads to the conclusion that the patterns of aging can only partially be attributed to the influence of a given variable. A multiple network of variables must be established in order to 'understand' the differences between different patterns of aging.

Considering the variability in our patterns due to the health factor, it is again necessary to distinghuish between results in which change or consistency might be better ascribed to the influence of other variables.

Patterns in which high scores are given regarding health as well as regarding the dimensions tested (attitude towards others, plan-making, anticipation of the future, etc.) or, vice versa, patterns in which low scores are found in both these sets of variables could point, again, to the dynamic aspect of a cognitive interpretation, assuming that the different dimensions were 'brought in congruence' by the predominance of the health factor. Such results occur in our cross-sectional findings (pp. 99, 104, 109) as well as in our longitudinal findings (pp. 99, 104). Opposite patterns with diverging scores in health and other dimensions emerge only twice (p. 99: high health scores, low life space scores; p. 109: low health scores, high life space scores). In these examples, other variables prove to have greater influence than health, thus underlining once more the necessity of embedding single results within the network of complex variables.

With respect to SES it is hardly possible to consider our findings as balanced, because the representatives of a 'higher' SES formed the majority in our longitudinal sample of 121 survivors. Therefore, these results should be noted, but not overinterpreted.

Contr. hum. Dev., vol. 3, pp. 113–126 (Karger, Basel 1976)

IX. Social Roles and Contacts in Old Age: Consistency and Patterns of Change

Erhard Olbrich and Ursula Lehr

Within the last 20 years, aging has emerged as a growing area of study. Within it, viewpoints and accents showed a shift. While research on biosomatic processes used to predominate, aging has come to be viewed more and more as a social problem rather than a biological or even a chronological one.

Today, we can observe a considerable amount of research on social role activities of the elderly. Part of this was stimulated by statements concerning a general isolation of the aged. There is a strong current of opinion saying that the fast pace of change in modern urban-industrial societies created serious obstacles to an effective social adjustment of old people, obstacles which render them 'incompetent', not only socially, but psychologically and personally as well (*Atchley,* 1972, p. 229). Students of old age involved in social action and social welfare seemed particularly inclined to add emphasis to their appeals to public opinion by alarming reports of the segregation or the isolation of the aged from present-day society (*Lehr and Rudinger,* 1969). It seems to have withdrawn increasingly from its older members since World War II. As a labor force, they are no longer sought, nor is their experience or wisdom appreciated by younger persons (*Atchley,* 1972, p. 129). Older people somehow seem to be left on their own, particularly with regard to the position they used to hold, which, of course, effects resultant feelings of being needed, as well as life satisfaction.

Interest in relationships between social role activities and aging was strongly aroused by the publication of *Cumming and Henry's* (1961) disengagement theory. According to this theory, isolation is not to be regarded just as a fate imposed by chronological aging. It rather appears as a result of a two-way process, one aspect of which may be described as a 'thinning out of the number of members in the social structure surrounding the individual, a diminishing of interaction with these members, and a restructuring of the goals of the systems' (*Newell,* 1961, p. 37). This is one half of the mutual withdrawal of society and older people, referred to as societal disengagement. The other part of disengagement obviously is initiated by the individual's own tendency to reduce social participation. This is viewed as a more or less inevitable, intrinsic process, which yields more personal satisfaction to the aged persons. The assumption underlying this conception seems to be, as *Atchley* (1972, p. 221) poignantly put it, that disengagement 'is both natural and good' at this stage of development.

Theory of Role Change

The most important contribution of disengagement theory to gerontology can be seen in the shift of psychological research from aspects of achievement and psychomotor skills to problems of social integration of the aged. *Parsons,* in his foreword to the book, certainly was right in predicting that the study of *Cumming and Henry* (1961) 'will serve as the most important focus of discussion of the problems on this level for some time'. In the decade and a half since its publication many studies were started concerning change in social participation with increasing age. Apparently, the theory itself changed (or was modified) with the ongoing years. And if there was one disengagement theory in 1961, we may distinguish at least seven (or more?) variations of it today.

(1) *Cumming and Henry* (1961) postulated a close relationship between lower social role activity (or participation) of the aged and higher life satisfaction, seen as an indicator of successful aging (the same relationship was seen between social role activity and a lower degree of satisfaction).

(2) This restriction of social role activity was explained by *Henry* in 1964 with his concept of 'intrinsic disengagement', which postulates 'disengagement with environment and engagement with self'.

(3) *Neugarten et al.* (1965) stressed the more qualitative aspects of involvement. They emphasized the fact that in some cases lower role activity can be associated with a higher degree of involvement within roles.

(4) *Havighurst and Neugarten* pointed to individual differences regarding the relationship between activity in social roles and life satisfaction. An individual revealing a certain specific personality structure may get a higher degree of satisfaction through lower social activity.

(5) Furthermore, special areas of engagement and disengagement were distinguished and the concepts of 'compensatory engagement' and 'selective disengagement-engagement' were introduced. The meaning of these concepts can easily be clarified. Around the age of 65 a man will, e. g., reduce his activity in the worker or the colleague role. At the same time he may show an increase of role activities within his family.

(6) With regard to the relevance of areas of high social actitivies for the individual, the pervading nature of disengagement processes was rather broadly questioned. Authors like *Havighurst* (1964), *Maddox* (1964) and *Palmore* (1968) stressed the observation that 'maintaining or developing substantial levels of

physical, mental and social activity is usually necessary for successful aging' (*Palmore,* 1969c, p. 58). Such conceptualizations were further developed by proponents of an actitivy theory of aging.

(7) Positions like these look incompatible with disengagement theory. We could, however, propose an integration of these divergent views using information from three age-groups: men, aged 50–55 (i. e. 10–15 years before retirement), men aged 60–65 (about retirement age), and men between 70 and 75 years.

The correlations between activity and satisfaction scores significantly differentiated these three groups and pointed to a sequence of engagement, disengagement (at the time of retirement), and reengagement (after adjustment to retirement). Those men, aged 60–65, who felt dissatisfied with retirement (and also those with a negative attitude toward approaching retirement), perceived the feeling of being needed and an overall higher activity as unpleasant. Only for this age group could we find a high correlation between higher social role activity and lower satisfaction. This result coincides with the disengagement theory and can be seen as a confirmation of it. Results of the age group 70–75 years, however, are contrary to the disengagement theory. Those men who show a higher role activity and who have more social contacts are more satisfied with their general life situation.

Further longitudinal studies, covering longer periods of life, should answer the question whether disengagement theory is applicable to some areas of social interaction and to a short period of the aging process only, or if it is descriptive of a more general developmental process. Stressing a psychologist's point of view which takes into account behavior as well as its cognitive representation, one could imagine that periods of transition – like retirement, which occurs during the years *Cumming and Henry* (1961) observed, but also like adolescence and other periods in life, characterized by the necessity of adaptions – require some sort of 'restriction', a kind of concentration on the internal process going on in order to cope with the new situation. Understood in this sense, disengagement might be perceived as one form of the person's reaction to the stress brought about by a different situation and a reorientation the individual has to make. Although there are many individual differences in reactions to stress (*Lazarus,* 1963, 1966), 'temporary disengagement', in our opinion, seems to be a frequent way of coping with the problems of some specific life situations throughout the course of life, but especially in old age.

Methodological Problems

We have seen that results of studies concerned with problems of role change and satisfaction with change do not lead in one direction. This may in part be due to methodological problems, some of which are relevant to the study of development.

(1) Most frequently, data from cross-sectional studies are used. Their interpretation may lead to confounding the variance caused by chronological change with the variance between samples. In longitudinal studies this source of error can be avoided, since each subject serves as his own control, thereby allowing developmental processes to be analyzed as they occur. Interpretation of longitudinal studies should be approached cautiously, however, with an eye for time of measurement effects and other sources of error pertaining to designs which involve repeated measures and some kind of control over intermediate influences on the subjects. (*Campbell and Stanley,* 1963).

(2) Furthermore, it seems to be necessary to approach problems of social change in a multidimensional way, taking account of biosomatic, personal, biographic, social and ecological variables. Relations of these variables to an increase or decrease in social role activities and to the individual's satisfaction or dissatisfaction have to be accounted for.

The present study is an attempt to describe longitudinally the development of older people's social role behavior and its cognitive and emotional appraisal over a period of 5 years. It will offer some cross-sectional comparisons as well as comparisons between older women and men. Moreover, it will show how activities in social roles and satisfaction with them are embedded in the total personal, biosomatic, ecological and social life space. Some attempts will be made to explain how variables from the whole life space of the individual functionally influence his social role behavior.

Our data were collected as a part of the Bonn Longitudinal Study on Aging (BLSA) which is described in detail by *Schmitz-Scherzer* in this volume (chap. X). As a sample, we chose 144 women and men whose social role behavior had been rated at the first, the third and the fourth measurement points (MPs) of the study. This was done after an extensive interview which followed a schedule originally developed by *Havighurst* and his co-workers. Full information about the interview schedule and the scales used for rating is given in the cross-national research report on 'Adjustment to retirement' by *Havighurst et al.* (1969). Ratings of social role behavior followed the proposition that an individual will engage differently in various areas of his social life space, thereby displaying a differentiated picture of his performance in various social roles. These areas of social interaction or life roles were analyzed and rather precisely delineated. These delineations, together with the more precise definitions of nine-point rating scales, were used as measures of activity and satisfaction (understood as an affective reflection of the actual role activity). The rating scales were generally considered to represent a continuum ranging from no activity to high activity and from negative to positive affect. Five points on the scales were anchored verbally. Measures in the following social roles were obtained: parents, grandparents, spouse, kin, friend, acquaintance, neighbor, club member and citizen. The subjects were not rated in their roles as workers, church members, homemakers and in their leisure time role, since these did not apply to the age group under consideration in the social and cultural context of Germany.

It is agreed that an assessment of this kind depends on clear and distinct definitions of the aspects of behavior under consideration, as well as on a standard type of measurable behavioral information from which ratings can go out. We attempted to bear this in mind during the study. Moreover, interviewers and raters were very carefully trained. A study on inter-rater agreement by *Fröhlich et al.* (1969, p. 23) showed that measures of activity obtained in the first follow-up session offered 'a reliable base' even for cross-national inferences, while satisfaction scores were 'of a more or less tentative nature'.

Estimates of reliability using *Heise*'s (1972) technique to check true-score instability of repeated measures and measurement errors yielded the following results for our data: The broad range of these coefficients will have implications for the interpretation of our results, indicating caution in the analysis of satisfaction scores of roles in social fields more peripheral to the individual, but allowing confidence in the results gained for activity scores in the more central social fields.

Results

Patterns of Activity and Satisfaction Scores

In a first attempt to form hypotheses about the simplest structure of the data under consideration, six factor analyses were computed, using activity and satisfaction scores measured at MPs I, III and IV of the study. Not too much space will be spent here on detailed reports of these analyses. It suffices to say that they had to be based on rather small percentages of common variance between ratings. Correlations between activity scores, which had been converted to Fisher z coefficients for purposes of averaging, had a mean of $r = 0.12$. The corresponding values for satisfaction scores reached a mean of $r = 0.15$. Linearity of relationship was established.

Two factors of role activity could be extracted from the ratings, one loading intrafamily role activities (parent and grandparent roles), the other those roles which indicate interactions with persons close to the aged individual (friend and acquaintance role). Comparisons of factor structures (*Fischer and Roppert,* 1964) yielded coefficients indicating a high similarity between these two factors over the whole span of observation.

Analysis of satisfaction scores showed analogous results. Two factors were consistently to be extracted, one concerning satisfaction with interactions with one's own offspring (parent and grandparent roles) and a second one, which can

Table I. Reliabilities of ratings of the social roles

Role	Activity	Satisfaction
Parent	0.92	0.66
Grandparent	0.88	0.42
Spouse	0.72	0.99
Neighbor	0.38	0.93
Friend	0.58	0.53
Acquaintance	0.35	0.26
Kin	0.50	0.19
Club member	0.44	0.53
Citizen	0.67	0.11
Median	0.58	0.53

Table II. Medians of activity and satisfaction ratings and results of ipsative comparisons between successive measurements[1]

	Medians at MPs			Comparisons between MPs		
	I	III	IV	I–III	III–IV	I–IV
Role activity						
Parent	6.89	7.00	6.46		ff	f
Grandparent	6.06	6.03	5.55			
Spouse	6.36	6.68	6.44	rr		
Neighbor	5.70	4.98	4.44	ff	ff	ff
Friend	4.91	4.97	3.55		ff	ff
Acquaintance	5.52	5.67	5.24	r	ff	
Kin	3.56	3.58	3.27		ff	
Club member	2.50	2.29	1.72	f		ff
Citizen	2.31	2;79	2.30		ff	f
Satisfaction						
Parent	7.41	7.44	7.20			f
Grandparent	7.30	7.52	7.21			
Spouse	7.04	7.55	7.42	r	f	
Neighbor	7.97	8.58	7.70	r	ff	f
Friend	7.87	7.33	7.07			f
Acquaintance	7.53	7.88	7.17		ff	
Kin	6.97	7.05	6.28		ff	ff
Club member	8.62	7.77	7.70	f		
Citizen	7.18	7.64	6.72		ff	

1 rr = rising of scores significant at $\alpha \leqq 0.01$; r = rising significant at $\alpha \leqq 0.05$; ff = falling of scores significant at $\alpha \leqq 0.01$; f = falling significant at $\alpha \leqq 0.05$.

be interpreted as a factor of satisfaction with interactions between the individual and psychologically close persons (friend and acquaintance).

More important than this information about hypothetical dimensions underlying the rated variables is the result that there was little common variance between ratings in the nine social roles. This seems to indicate that nine different segments of behavior were measured which deserve a more differentiated analysis.

Change in Activity and Satisfaction Scores

Another step in our endeavor to find out if the subjects had changed their social role behavior over time was to use Wilcoxon's matched-pair signed-ranks test, which allowed for ipsative comparisons of scores older persons had received in successive years of the study. Tests were run for the nine parameters of activity and satisfaction separately. The results are presented in table II, which, in addition, gives medians of the subjects scores, describing central tendencies in the measures of the whole sample. Comparing these over time, of course, need not necessarily parallel the results indicated by the more appropriate Wilcoxon T indices, upon which our further descriptions rely.

A glance at table II shows that our subjects were remarkably active in their intrafamilial roles (parent, grandparent and spouse). Changes in these roles activities in social fields somewhat more peripheral to the individual.

While role activities in the parent role increased during the first 3 years of our study, and then decreased, those in the grandparent role showed no significant change at all. Activities indicating interactions with one's spouse rose and fell during our period of observation. There was no significant change between the beginning and the end of the 4-year interval.

A glance at table II shows that our subjects were remarkably active in their intrafamilial roles (parent, grandparent and spouse). Changes in these roles were not as frequent or as marked as those observed for role activities in social fields somewhat more peripheral to the individual.

Overall changes were not so marked in these fields of interaction whose central importance to the individual made them obviously worth a consistent and rather high amount of activity. A general decrease of role activity was registered in fields of the social life space that can be considered more peripheal. From table II one can see that all changes – aside from a growth of activity in the acquaintance role during the first 3 years of our study – indicated decreasing role activities. There should not be too many inferences drawn from this, since reliabilities of the ratings tend to be rather low.

Table II also gives evidence that changes in role activities were, in general, paralleled by changes in satisfaction with these activities. This point will be extended and made more precise later. Something has to be said here, however, about the general tendency of change of satisfaction scores alone, which are decreasing. It will be noted that medians of the respective role ratings were rather high throughout the study, i. e. the aged persons in our sample usually associated a high degree of experienced positive affect with all role activities. So there is evidence in our data that satisfaction decreases with decreasing role activities, especially in fields more peripheral to the individual. But the remaining levels of satisfaction are still so high that one cannot infer any suffering from social isolation for our men and women in their sixties and seventies.

We have analyzed consistencies and changes in the same way for the following subgroups of our sample separately, for women and men, and for the younger (born between 1900 and 1905) and the older cohort (born between 1890 and 1895). There is not enough space here to give the full details of results gained in these analyses, but we can report in just a few words about the most important facts. There was somewhat more change in social activities for men than for women, and there was more change in the older group than in the younger one. But while the overall direction of change, denoting a decrease in activities, was more marked for men than for women, differences between the two age groups were of another kind. Our results showed no change of activity for the younger cohort when MPs I and III were compared longitudinally. Decreases of activity scores in peripheral social areas were noted only when later follow-ups were included in the analyses. Compared to the younger group, subjects of the older sample also changed role activities during the first part of the study. They increased social interactions with spouses, while activities as neighbors and club members were decreasing.

All the other changes in both cohorts were characterized by falling scores. There was just one exception on this. The older group even increased interactions with spouses between the first and the fourth MP.

The overall impression one gets from these differentiated analyses is that the women group and, to a certain extent, the younger cohort show less change and only contribute in the later years of the study to the decrease in social interaction. The question, of course, remains to be answered, if this means just a delay or a principally different pattern of role change in the social field.

It should be added that the women subgroup and the younger cohort showed no change of satisfaction with intrafamilial role activities. This seems to indicate that they were not aware of any change in affective appraisal of these social relations. These subgroups' satisfaction scores in the extrafamilial roles, in general, again paralleled their role activity measures.

In addition to these longitudinal analyses, cross-sectional comparisons were made using the Mann-Whitney U test, which can be regarded as a generalization of the Wilcoxon T test for independent samples (*Wilcoxon,* 1945). From 27 comparisons between activity scores of the younger and older cohort (nine roles in three follow-ups of the study), only two were significant at $\alpha \leqslant 0.05$. The younger subjects of our sample were more active in their kin role, at both MPs I and III. None of the 27 corresponding tests of cross-sectional differences between satisfaction scores gave a result significant at the 5-percent level of significance.

This seems remarkable. While longitudinal analyses, using each subject for his own comparison, came up with rather detailed results, indicating consistencies as well as processes of change over a 5-year period, cross-sectional studies of two subgroups of the same sample, one 10 years younger than the other, showed nearly no change, let alone a process. Although one will have to take account of errors of measurement, one cannot avoid stating that intracohort variation in these cross-sectional comparisons seems to have covered intergroup variation.

Combined Analyses of Activity and Satisfaction

In addition to such longitudinal and cross-sectional analyses of single parameters, combinations of these seemed relevant in order to answer psychologically more meaningful questions. Our intention was to analyze differences in role activity together with differences in satisfaction, i. e. indices of change in overt role behavior and the subjects' affective appraisals of them. So, for each of the fields of social behavior, we formed four groups from our sample. Two of these were characterized by congruent changes of activity and satisfaction in the respective roles. In group one, both parameters, activity and satsifaction, increased (A+, S+); in the second, they both decreased (A–, S–). The remaining two groups were characterized by divergent changes of the individual's behavior and their affective appraisal, i. e. in groups three and four increasing role activity was combined with decreasing satisfaction (A+, S–), and decreasing activity with increasing satisfaction (A–, S+).

Comparing these groups over all fields of social interaction (two-by-two χ^2-test) gave evidence of highly significant differences. The number of aged persons showing congruent changes was significantly larger than those of subjects who were aware of an affective appraisal divergent from their manifest social activities. These differences became especially apparent between the first and fourth and between the third and fourth MPs.

More specific tests of these changes, taking account of single roles only, showed the following results. In the parent, kin, friend, and spouse roles, there were significantly more older persons with congruent change of role behavior and its subjective appraisal. Besides these statistically significant results, there were similar tendencies in all the remaining social fields.

In extension of these combined analyses which compare patterns of congruent and divergent change, especially two subgroups were considered. Group A was made up of those subjects whose role activity decreased with age while their satisfaction increased. This is the kind of change that would be expected by proponents of disengagement theory. As a contrast, an ideal group according to

Table III. Combined analyses of change in activity and satisfaction[1]

Roles	Number of aged persons showing the following patterns of change throughout the time of the BLSA				Differences (χ^2-test)	
	A– S+ (group A)	A+ S+ (group B)	A+ S–	A– S–	between all groups	between group A and B
Parent	28	38	28	16	3.94[2]	1.23
Grandparent	30	48	28	33	1.23	3.71
Kin	52	84	43	58	3.88[2]	7.01[3]
Friend	37	78	29	49	4.69[2]	13.91[3]
Acquaintance	43	82	40	63	1.17	11.55[3]
Neighbor	30	87	50	43	0.25	26.80[3]
Club member	23	64	33	26	1.78	18.39[3]
Spouse	24	46	7	47	5.81[2]	6.30[2]
Citizen	37	62	47	41	0.19	5.82[2]
	304	589	305	376 [3]	17.81[3]	90.32[3]

1 A+ = Increasing role activity; A– = decreasing role activity; S+ = increasing satisfaction; S– = decreasing satisfaction.
2 χ^2 significant at $\alpha \leqq 5\%$.
3 χ^2 significant at $\alpha \leqq 1\%$.

notions of activity theory was selected (group B). It consisted of subjects who combined rising role activity with increasing satisfaction in their development.

Comparisons of these groups showed that in all roles there were more individuals belonging to group B than A. This means that persons who disengaged socially were in the minority in all social roles. Throughout the social life space, older subjects whose pattern of change coincided with activation theory prevailed. Differences in simple χ^2-tests were significant in all fields of social behavior, with exceptions only in the parent and grandparent roles. These were the roles with rather high ratings in the first year of the study. Table III gives more precise data on these results. According to these findings, the development of older persons' social role behavior shows a tendency toward more congruency between overt activity in the social field and its inner appraisal. Of course, changes of the kind described by disengagement theory do exist, but they represent one form of development which is hidden behind that described by a congruent affective representation of manifest social interaction. We cannot analyze how the subjects in our sample came to develop congruency or discrepancy, disengagement or increasing activation. We can only offer a first approach to a functional analysis of change in activity and satisfaction.

Functional Analyses of Change in Activity and Satisfaction

Again we distinguished between persons characterized by congruent or divergent patterns of change. In addition to these, we considered subjects who did not change in one or both of the role parameters. Proceeding in this way, we could divide our whole sample into nine subgroups that were arranged in a three-by-three two-factorial design. The factors 'role activity' and 'satisfaction' had steps indicating increase, no change, and decrease over time. Into the cells of this design we read data that had been assessed in the first year of the BLSA. These were biosomatic variables like vital capacity, a rating of the subject's general physical state, measures of blood pressure, measures of cardiovascular insufficiency, and ratings of sight, hearing, and of the degree of physical mobility. In addition, we also analyzed social data, namely the subject's formal education, his family status, the number of persons living in his household, the number of his grandchildren, and his age. A third group of variables was made up of psychological data: attitudes towards other persons, satisfaction with one's present life situation, sense of being needed, the degree of achieved congruency between vocational goals and their realization, outlook toward the future and plans for the future, concern for one's own physical well-being, concern for the preservation of one's social life space, sense of a threatening restriction, and finally, intelligence. The hypothesis seemed justified that if systematic differences were to be found between these earliest measures of biosomatic, social, and psychological data, these could be assumed to have functionally determined changes in role activity and satisfaction.

On the whole, 414 analyses of variance were run to localize those variables which had influenced changes in the nine roles between MP I and MP III and between MP I and MP IV. To summarize their results here at least very roughly, we have to state that changes in parameters of intrafamilial roles were influenced primarily by variables characterizing an individual's immediate social situation, like his family status, the number of his grandchildren, or the number of persons living in his household. The second class of variables influencing intrafamilial role change were those describing the individual's own biosomatic condition, above all his blood pressure, sight, and general physical state.

On the other hand, changes in extrafamilial role activity and satisfaction seemed to be influenced primarily by those variables we refer to here as psychological ones. Especially the congruence of an aged person's vocational goals and their realization, his attitude toward others, his attitude toward the future, his sense of being needed, and his concern for the preservation of his social life space seemed systematically related to changes in the individual's more peripheral roles. The characteristic common to all these variables is that they indicate cognitively represented facts. We can state that changes even in rather peripheral social roles are co-determined by a person's awareness of his psychological situation.

Summary and Discussion

Changes in his life situation no doubt require an aging individual to adapt his behavior – be it manifestly or in affective or cognitive reactions – to the new stages of his development. The present study is an attempt to analyze social role activities as well as satisfaction with them in 144 older people belonging to two cohorts about 10 years apart in age.

The major results were gained from longitudinal comparisons; better than cross-sectional ones, they gave evidence of a rather differentiated pattern of consistencies and changes in the field of social interactions. With varying age, this pattern varies in specific ways in the single areas defined by single social roles. Ipsative comparisons, i. e. comparisons over time with each individual serving as his own control, gave results indicative of the processes going on in this development. This certainly goes a long way to support our study. We have to admit some serious weaknesses, however, the most important of which is a sampling error. Selective dropout of the subjects and selective survival (cf. chap. X) will bias our results. Their interpretation has to be restricted insofar as generalizations can be made only to a selected part of the age group. Nevertheless, we had a chance to observe development as it occurred. This defintely has an advantage over cross-sectional techniques, which not only are subject to the danger of sampling errors, but can make comparisons between samples only as far as whole groups are concerned. They usually have to deal with an error term arising from the pooled variance of individual differences. Direct regard and analysis of intrasubject variation are impossible to them. Moreover, they contaminate development effects with generational differences. This seems to be the most important point to be made. Of course, we are aware of possible influential test effects or instrumental decay. *Rudinger* deals more comprehensively with these effects and with techniques to control them throughout the period of data collection and statistical analysis in the BLSA.

In our approach to a functional analysis of changes in social role behavior we have checked the effects of 23 variables. This, in our opinion, is a mere first step toward a more complex form of analysis of the development process. It will have to be expanded and further forms of multivariate analysis tried out. Besides these plans for more sophisticated data analysis we see another necessity for longitudinal research. What we are missing is an effective control over, or even observations of, intermediate influences on the subjects' behavior between measurements. The use of techniques known from field experimentation and from controlled variation of independent variables might become fruitful extensions of longitudinal research designs.

Although our study leaves many methodological questions unanswered and many wishes unfulfilled, we think it is useful to bring the results together with some prior knowledge and thereby find some evidence of patterns of social development in advanced age. To sum up some results very roughly, we noticed considerable stability in intrafamilial social interaction, especially in interaction with one's own children and grandchildren. We also noted more dynamic change in roles rather peripheral to the psychological self. Regarding social role behavior in its overt manifestation (activity) and in its affective representation (satisfaction) at the same time, we could look at overt and inner processes, catching a glimpse of forms and degrees of their congruence or divergence. Our impression is that changes occurring can ce conceptualized as forms of adapting to and coping with developmental tasks in *Havighurst's* (1956) sense. Levels and kinds of activities of our group match the physical, social, and individual conditions of older people's life in a meaningful way. There is a great amount of interindividual variance in social role behavior, which means that there is a broad range of individual variation within this general framework of adaptation.

Predominant in our sample is a form of adaptation characterized by congruence between changes in role activities and satisfaction with them. The tendency toward congruence between these parameters of role behavior became even more evident in later follow-ups of our research.

Regarding such processes, we think that those changes described by *Cumming and Henry's* (1961) disengagement theory play a minor role in the development of older people's social role behavior. We prefer to follow *Secord and Backman's* (1964) theoretical view of the changes going on when an individual is urged to adapt to a new situation in his development. According to the authors, the individual may be pressured by circumstances which we might find to be physical, biological, psychological, or social ones, to change. But he will tend not to appreciate divergance or even discrepancy between his behavior and its cognitive representation. What *Secord and Backman* (1964, p. 584) stress is the fact that an individual will actively attempt to maintain stability of self and behavior; faces with a changing situation, the individual 'actively uses techniques or mechanisms for maintaining his interpersonal environment so as to maximize congruency'.

Now the general conviction seems to be that, in age and old age, changes in social behavior more or less impinge upon an individual from the outside, forcing themselves upon him, so that he can only react in order to maintain the above mentioned stability between 'inside and outside'. Results of our study do not fully support this view. They indicate that even performance in social roles more peripheral to the individual is influenced by central cognitive and affective aspects.

Similarly, correlational studies show that intrafamilial roles are embedded in a background charcterized by variables very close to the individual, like, e. g., his own biosomatic situation, his personal ecological and social environment, etc. (*Olbrich,* 1975). This is the background on which an aging individual bases his actions, and which he generally includes rather competently when acting in his intrafamilial roles.

We do not wish to forget those aged individuals who internally represent changes in social interaction differently from their overt manifestations. These are the aged persons reacting in ways the disengagement theory proposed.

It is difficult for a psychologist to understand these forms of reaction and to interpret them. Looking at the work of theorists in personality psychology such as *Lazarus* (1963, 1966), one is led to assume that a discrepancy between role activity and satisfaction with it will scarcely be preserved for a long time. According to these notions it will be hard to live with inner representations of one's behavior completely different from or even contradictory to its actual realizations. Results of our study confirm what experiences in counseling and psychotherapy (*Rogers,* 1973) have shown to be a helpful process: a tendency towards establishing a congruent relationship between psychological self and experience of one's own behavior as well as one's environment. Our data even make us aware of the change an aging individual experiences. He can actively introduce change in his social behavior on the basis of affective and cognitive appraisals of his perceived social situation, and, even more important, of his personal situation.

Contr. hum. Dev., vol. 3, pp. 127–136 (Karger, Basel 1976)

X. Longitudinal Change in Leisure Behavior of the Elderly

R. Schmitz-Scherzer

The number of publications dealing with leisure behavior among aging people is increasing rapidly. Activities termed as leisure behavior are generally engaged in voluntarily, without any particular outside pressure. The extent of interest and involvement in such activity has a lot to do with how elderly persons spend their time, which makes the growing scientific attention to the area of leisure behavior understandable. Of course, the growth of research in this area is also related to current concern with the development of public and private programs for the aged, a topic also encountered in scientific journals. Thus, proponents of socially engaged psychological intervention emphasize the importance of daily activity and leisure activity in their attempts to institute acceptance of continuing activity in old age as a public norm (*Lehr,* 1972). Leisure activity also plays a role in rehabilitation programs for the elderly (*Schmitz-Scherzer,* 1970). Analyses of leisure activity certainly are of significance for adult education programs. Offers intended to promote information and civic know-how, develop mental and physical potential, and encourage social interaction as well as recreation reach more people when they take the target group's everyday habits into consideration (*Becker,* 1974; *Haag,* 1974; *Orbens,* 1974). The agencies responsible for planning public policy are already demanding 'need-oriented' program development, thereby raising the question of guidelines to be used in identifying the determinants of everyday and leisure behavior (*Kühn and Plagemann,* 1974).

Previous studies have addressed themselves to the description of leisure behavior among aging people and to certain traditional determining variables such as socioeconomic status (*Kleemeier,* 1961; for an overview of the literature, see *Schmitz-Scherzer,* 1975c). Thus, *Blume* (1962) demonstrated the paramount connection between education and leisure behavior among older people, which are proportionally related to each other. The higher the level of education, the more diverse and numerous were the interests which found expression in elderly people's leisure behavior. Studies of this type often fail to disentangle the effects of closely interrelated socioeconomic variables. High socioeconomic status usually has certain educational, vocational, and financial prerequisites. It hardly comes as a surprise when a study reports similar intensity and frequency of leisure behavior for those with higher education, better jobs, and higher income. However, these studies seldom yield insights relevant for planning purposes.

The occurrence of change in everyday behavior has been investigated less extensively (*Schmitz-Scherzer,* 1975a, b). This is a particularly crucial point, however, which would not only enable us to make scientifically founded statements on changes occurring among the adult population but would help us to answer questions about the behavioral possibilities of older people. Leisure is an important influence on adjustment to retirement or coming to terms with the fact that the children have grown up and left home. This line of investigation is followed by *Schmitz-Scherzer* (1969) who showed that totally new activities are seldom taken up in later life. Instead, there is more likely to be continued or extended activity in previously established areas. These cross-sectional results have yet to be longitudinally substantiated. The confirmation of these findings would be of value to those engaged in planning and carrying out programs for the aged.

This essay will submit a first analysis of the question of constancy and variability in leisure behavior. It is based on a study of the frequency of some selected leisure activities, which are not exhaustive or fully representative of the field of leisure time, but which do deal with activities which seem to be of importance within the framework of extensive gerontological questioning.

We are not referring here to the social contacts which were studied with methods proposed by *Havighurst et al.* (1969) for measuring certain social roles. This analysis will be presented in chapter xxx of this volume.

The frequency of engaging in the leisure time activities included in this analysis were rated on some 9- and some 6-point scales (0 = never, 1 = very seldom, up to 6 or 9 = very often, daily), according to information obtained on specific questions in a half-standardized interview.

Altogether the following spheres of action were referred to: paying visits, being visited, entertainment with other people, taking trips, going for a walk, going to the movies and going out for a drink or a meal, reading newspapers and magazines, gardening, listening to the radio, and watching television.

Results of a Cross-Sectional Analysis

The first inspection of these data was carried out by *Schmitz-Scherzer* (1969) in the form of a cross-sectional analysis. Besides describing the leisure activities of this age group, the main intention of this study was to indentify the determining variables of leisure time behavior. It turned out that the range and variety of leisure time activities of the aging and old people we were studying is by all means comparable to that of the younger generation. In the cross-sectional view there was no difference (of age) between men and women of the age of 60–65 and 70–75 years. On the contrary, the differences found in this comparison could be ascribed to the different social situation of the members of both age groups.

The younger ones were still active in their jobs, whereas the older persons had generally retired. Widowhood was found more often in the older group than in the younger one. From these results first hypotheses could be formed about the small relevance of chronological age as a determinant of old people's leisure time behavior, which could be demonstrated by *Schmitz-Scherzer and Stroedel* (1971) for other samples as well.

Nevertheless, social variables such as education, income, and occupational position were of decisive importance according to the results of these analyses. These variables which mostly serve as indirect evident for measuring social status, influenced leisure time behavior in the expected manner: the higher social status, education, income, and professional position were, the more distinctive and pronounced was the everyday behavior. With lower status, television, going for a walk, and reading newspapers were the most frequently mentioned activities; with higher status, many additional, more expensive activities and hobbies were added.

Beside these determining variables which could partly be anticipated on the basis of a study about the leisure time activities of younger people, the first analysis of these data gave further information about the defining quantities which so far had hardly been studied. It turned out that a bad state of health, as assessed by physicians, can reduce the extent of everyday activities considerably. According to these results, a bad state of health reduced not only the frequency of leisure time activities, but seems to diminish the number of such occupations generally.

To a certain extent, test values, e.g. IQ or measures of rigidity, also had considerable influence on the leisure time behavior, whereby more intelligent persons were more active and interested than less intelligent persons, and persons with a high degree of rigidity represented themselves as less active and resourceful in the field of leisure. These persons also made less use of information from printed media such as newspapers and books.

Attitude measures, such as attitude to other people, also showed an influence on leisure time behavior. The more positive one's attitude towards other persons is, the more social contacts, but also activities not bound to social contact, he shows. Moreover, activity as a formal characteristic of behavior seems to stimulate everyday activities insofar as persons, who show a certain general activity, realize many activities in this field (sector) of behavior.

The complex relational structure of leisure time behavior, personality, and situation shows that everyday behavior cannot be regarded in isolation from the individual and his situation.

Longitudinal Results

Beside the question of identifying the determinants of everyday behavior, it is important to ask whether they change and, if so, what are the determinants of these changes. Only few studies about these topics exist, but some preliminary work on these problems has begun (*Schmitz-Scherzer,* 1975a, b). The results presented in this essay are based on the methodological experiences gained from these studies. They depend on calculations of reliability and stability and on analyses of covariance for repeated measurement with the factors point of measurement, age and sex, and social status as the covariate, which were calculated after inspecting means and variance at the respective points of measurement.

Inspection of Means

Beside giving a first insight into the data, an inspection of the means can at most give a first glimpse of the answer to questions about the change in everyday behavior with growing age. Further statements need statistical confirmation, which will be taken up in the following passages.

The means of the data about everyday behavior (table I) almost without exception show little sign of distinguishable systematic change among the group of men. Only the frequencies of watching TV and reading a newspaper increase continuously over the period of investigation. The frequencies of paying visits and going to the pictures, on the other hand, show a continuous decrease. The frequency of churchgoing remains constant.

If the first point of investigation is compared with the fourth, only the average frequencies of short rides or excursions increase within the curves of the men group. A decrease of means appears in the average frequencies of gardening, being visited, entertainment with others, and going for a walk. The average frequency of listening to the radio and reading magazines also decreases. Only going out for a drink or a meal remains constant in a comparison of the first point of investigation with the fourth.

Summing up, we can say that in the men group the decrease in average of everyday activity frequencies predominates in spite of minor variability is considered. Only the frequency of watching TV and reading the newspapers increases slightly. Going out and the average frequency of churchgoing remain

Table I. Descriptive statistics for the men at all four measurement points

Variables	Measurement points							
	I		II		III		IV	
	mean	SD	mean	SD	mean	SD	mean	SD
Reading the newspaper	5.6	0.9	5.6	1.1	5.6	1.2	5.7	1.2
Gardening	2.8	0.5	1.8	0.9	1.7	1.0	2.0	0.9
Being visited	5.1	1.9	5.2	1.9	4.9	2.2	4.3	1.8
Paying visits	5.2	2.0	4.4	1.9	3.9	1.9	3.6	1.8
Entertainment with others	4.2	1.9	3.0	2.0	3.2	1.9	2.6	1.7
Going to the movies	1.9	0.9	0.3	0.7	0.3	0.7	0.2	0.5
Going out for a meal or a drink	3.9	3.1	4.2	2.7	4.3	2.5	3.9	2.8
Church attendance	3.7	2.5	3.7	2.8	3.7	2.8	3.7	2.9
Going for a walk	4.9	1.2	4.8	1.7	4.1	1.8	4.4	2.1
Excursions	2.3	1.3	2.5	1.5	2.3	1.4	2.7	1.6
Reading magazines	3.1	1.8	2.8	2.0	3.1	2.2	2.6	1.9
Radio	3.9	2.0	4.2	2.3	3.8	2.4	3.9	2.3
Television	4.1	2.5	5.0	1.8	5.3	1.4	5.6	1.3

nearly unchanged over the period of investigation. Yet it must be referred to the fact that these changes, too, still remain within the average range of the frequencies. A similar picture exists in the women group (table II). Here, too, a decrease of means can be identified in the changing mean values. Continuously proceeding decreases or increases are seldom to be observed. Only the average frequency of entertainment with others and going to the movies decreases continuously, that of watching television increases. Within the set of observed means, increases are found for the characteristics 'reading newspapers', 'gardening', and 'being visited', when the first and fourth investigation dates are compared. Beside the increase of average frequencies of 'going out', 'churchgoing', 'excursions' and 'reading magazines' are found on that basis. Decreases are found for 'paying visits', and 'going for a walk'. The frequency of 'listening to the radio' remains constant in this comparison. Here, too, all changes remain in the range of average frequencies (tables I, II).

Summing up, it must be pointed out that the decrease of the average frequencies of everyday activities is numerically very small in the women group, too, but that the indications of increase or constancy dominate. Certainly, they also do not appear continuously here, but they develop irregularly. The use of

Table II. Descriptive statistics for the women at all four measurement points

Variables	Measurement points							
	I		II		III		IV	
	mean	SD	mean	SD	mean	SD	mean	SD
Reading the newspaper	4.8	1.4	5.4	1.4	5.0	1.9	5.1	1.8
Gardening	1.4	0.6	1.6	1.1	1.2	1.2	2.3	1.6
Being visited	3.0	2.6	5.6	1.7	6.0	2.3	4.7	2.0
Paying visits	5.4	2.1	5.5	1.9	5.4	2.3	4.8	2.2
Entertainment with others	5.1	1.9	4.4	2.3	4.2	2.1	3.8	2.3
Going to the movies	2.3	1.5	0.6	0.9	0.5	1.2	0.3	0.9
Going out for a meal or a drink	3.4	2.4	3.6	2.2	4.0	2.0	3.6	2.7
Church attendance	2.0	1.6	3.9	3.0	3.9	3.0	3.5	3.0
Going for a walk	4.5	1.3	4.7	2.2	4.5	1.9	4.3	1.9
Excursions	2.3	1.6	3.2	1.7	2.6	1.3	2.7	1.7
Reading magazines	2.7	1.9	3.1	2.0	3.2	1.8	3.1	2.0
Radio	4.8	1.8	5.1	1.5	5.1	1.7	4.8	2.1
Television	3.1	2.3	4.4	2.1	4.8	1.6	5.1	1.8

communication media (TV, magazines, radio, newspaper) shows increasing average frequencies. A further analysis of data will show which trends can be confirmed.

Summing up the results of the inspection of means and variance of each turn of investigation it can be said: (a) The number of changes proceeding continuously in the sense of a continuous decrease or increase of the means over all points of measurement is rather small. Constancy predominates. (b) By far the most frequent kind of possible changes are courses. Over the different points of measurement means fall and/or rise more or less unsystematically, but they remain in the average range of each subject measured. (c) Comparing the first and fourth points of investigation we find reductions in the sense of a reduction of the means very often. They make up three fifths of all changes, which can be stated in this way, but they move within the average range of frequencies. (d) A large proportion of the changes indicated here depend in part on very small differences between means. Most of them can possibly not be statistically confirmed. (e) Generally, the average frequency of leisure activities decreases, with the exception of the frequencies of watching TV and reading newspapers which increase slightly.

Table III. Reliabilities and stabilities of leisure data

Variables	Total sample		men		women	
	Reliability	Stability	Reliability	Stability	Reliability	Stability
Reading the newspaper	0.595	0.600	0.647	0.658	0.730	0.520
Gardening	0.364	0.998	0.496	0.999	0.192	0.922
Being visited	0.561	0.605	0.494	0.854	0.599	0.413
Paying visits	0.404	0.931	0.258	0.999	0.430	0.999
Entertainment with others	0.496	0.488	0.384	0.733	0.409	0.641
Going to the movies	0.448	0.141	0.431	0.171	0.491	0.170
Going out for a meal or a drink	0.635	0.999	0.710	0.999	0.490	0.973
Church attendance	0.816	0.959	0.892	0.916	0.712	0.917
Going for a walk	0.403	0.782	0.462	0.327	0.391	0.873
Excursions	0.254	0.999	0.252	0.929	0.228	0.918
Reading magazines	0.626	0.357	0.902	0.161	0.386	0.887
Radio	0.541	0.968	0.534	0.923	0.505	0.863
Televison	0.694	0.433	0.999	0.054	0.459	0.999

Reliabilities and Stabilities

Heise 1972 proposes a model for calculating the reliabilities and stabilities of a measurement based on the correlations of a measurement over all points of measurement. As it is mentioned in chapter xxx of this volume, the stabilities calculated according to this model can provide some information about intra-individual changes insofar as they repeatedly compare the position of a single individual relative to the position of other individuals from measurement point to measurement point. In this connection it must be remembered that insufficient reliabilities can also be signs of changes (chap. x, p. xxx). In this context a coefficient of 0.60 and higher shall be considered as evidence of sufficient stabilities or reliabilities.

Measures which should record the frequency of leisure activities have sufficient reliability in only a few cases if the total group is considered. Accordingly, those measures have only little reliability. Stability can be found to a greater extent considering the total group. In other words, there are hints of stabilities of some measurements over the period of investigation (table III), but they are often accompanied by insufficient reliabilities.

More specifically, the total group shows sufficient reliability for length of day, frequency of going out, churchgoing, and frequency of reading magazines and watching TV. The measures gardening, frequency of going out, and churchgoing signalize stabilities with sufficient reliabilities. A hint at changes accompanied by sufficient reliabilities is found only for length of day and frequency of watching TV. All the other measures are not reliable and hint at changes or stability.

In the group of men, stability with sufficient reliability is found for length of day, frequency of going out, and churchgoing. Changes with sufficient reliability are indicated for frequency of reading magazines. In the group of women only the frequency of churchgoing presents stability with sufficient reliability, and changes are found for the frequency of reading newspapers. On the whole, small reliabilities must be referred to in this connection. Sufficient stabilities are found in about 50% of the data pool. Following our convention, only frequency of churchgoing is reliable throughout all groups. In all groups, gardening, frequency of paying visits, going out, churchgoing, taking excursions, and watching TV are stable (table III).

Summing up, we can say that our data show sex differences with regard to the stabilities and reliabilities of some variables. Only length of day and frequency of churchgoing are generally reliable, only gardening, paying visits, going out, churchgoing, and frequency of excursions are generally stable.

Results of the Analysis of Variance

The analysis of covariance, which is reported on in the following statements, included the factors points of measurement, age (60–69 versus persons aged 70 or above) and sex, and, as covariate, social status (in these analyses). Our measurements show no significant interactions. More visits are paid by women ($M = 5.7–4.9$; $F = 18.9$; $p < 0.001$). 8% of the total variance of this variable is based on sex. The factor point of measurement discriminates only a few variables of this data pool. 3.9–60. 8% of the total variance are based on this factor for some variables. The frequency of reading the newspaper and watching TV changed in the course of the investigation time ($F = 175.8$ and 31.3, $p < 0001$ % in both cases; declared variance 60.8 and 12.7%). The indicated changes proceed according to the means in the sense of increasing frequency ($M = 4.9–5.7$, and 3.6–5.5) from the first to the last point of measurement). The frequency of gardening also changes during the period of investigation ($F = 10.6$; $p < 0.001$% for 5.3% declared variance). In the course of the investigation, an increase of frequency of gardening is to be seen ($M = 1.7–2.1$). The frequency of being visited and entertainment also shows changes ($F = 7.3$ and 8.4, both $p < 0.001$% for 2.9 and 3.9% declared variance). The means show a distinct reduction during the period of investigation with 5.3–4.6 and 4.4–3.2, respectively, whereby an undulating pattern was observed. The adjustment of the social status does not alter our results based on covariance.

Summary and Discussion

The discussion of the results in question has to proceed from the following main results: (1) Hints at constancy predominate. More than 50% of the activities which were analyzed by us show neither group-specific nor intraindividual changes. (2) Differences of reliabilities and stabilities between the sex groups in their contents refer to different intraindividual patterns of change in the sex groups. The frequency of being visited, for example, remains stable among the men, but not among the women, who show a stable frequency of going for walks over the period of measurement. Reading newspapers is stable only in the group of men, whereas in the group of women only frequency of reading magazines and watching TV remains stable. The only variables that are stable throughout both sex groups in the sense that they lack intraindividual changes are the frequency of excursions, going out, and gardening, as well as frequency of churchgoing and paying visits. (3) Opposite to this distinct intraindividual variability, possibly indicated by the not quite sufficient coefficients of reliability – especially considering the high uncertainty of the measurements – stand only a few group-specific changes, which could be found in the analysis of variance. Reading newspapers as well as frequency of watching TV and gardening increase, being visited and entertainment with others decrease. All changes have an undulating pattern, which means that the means of our measurement rise and fall seemingly unsystematically over all points of measurement, which otherwise remain within the average range of each frequency. The constancy of frequencies of everyday activities, which was also found in the longitudinal study and which is given to a great extent in both group-specific and intraindividual forms, may be surprising at first, since it seems to admit an influence of the variable chronological age *per se* only in a few cases.

But also those hints at changes of some everyday activities which are numerically rather small can be interpreted as an indication of a reduction of frequencies, which increases with age and with which corresponding activities are performed, since the intensification found in the group-specific investigation of use of media, and gardening as well as reduction of being visited and entertainment with others must be considered under different aspects in the context of the results of gerontological investigation.

It must, for example, be kept in mind, that precisely in the 6th and 7th life decade a great number of social changes come into existence. Both retirement and children's departure from home may bring about an extensive change of the everyday situation. This may lead to a reduction of certain contacts. *Schmitz-Scherzer* (1975a, b) demonstrated that family-related contacts will be intensified; extrafamilial contacts will partly be reduced. At the same time, the use of the mass media is intensified according to our results. This seems to be less explainable with *Havighurst*'s (1963) modified disengagement theory, according to which a part of the social contacts will be intensified at the cost of others, but it seems more likely to be explainable as a reaction to a changing situation. After all, our material shows too few hints at group-specific changes in the sense of increase or decrease of activity frequencies. The results predominantly showing constancy refer rather to an extreme stability. Therefore, the increased attention to communication media cannot be interpreted as increasing passivity. In that case a decrease should also have been found for some other activities.

The changes, which we presented in an interindividual approach, point to the existence of a greater number of individual variations which could be demonstrated with the calculation of the coefficients of stability according to *Heise* (1971). The inspection of the means also shows such variabilities from measurement point to measurement point. These changes may therefore be attributed largely to determining variables, which are intrinsic to the individual and his given situation. Our cross-sectional analyses (*Schmitz-Scherzer,* 1969) have shown the complex pattern of determinants of everyday activities. This leads to the conclusion that the most relevant variables are situational, social, economic, hygienic, and psychological variables and that chronological age has little significance for the explication of our results.

In any case we have no (there is no) general model of age to integrate our results. On the other hand, our results suggest an ability of regulation, which is shown to a high degree by the persons in our study and thereby clearly demonstrated the ability to react adequately and actively to changes in their surroundings according to their abilities and possibilities.

Contr. hum. Dev., vol. 3, pp. 137–146 (Karger, Basel 1976)

XI. Survivors and Nonsurvivors - Two Fundamental Patterns of Aging

U. Lehr and R. Schmitz-Scherzer

Longevity as an Interdisciplinary Problem

Growing interest in topics contrasting survivors and nonsurvivors is evident in longitudinal studies of longevity or life expectancy. A number of longitudinal aging research projects have been examined from the standpoint of survivor-nonsurvivor differences, such as the Normative Aging Study of Boston Veterans (*Rose and Bell,* 1971), the Duke Longitudinal Study of Aging (*Palmore and Jeffers,* 1971; *Busse,* 1969; *Pfeiffer,* 1969 and follow-up data from the Bethesda Study (*Birren et al.,* 1963b), analyzed in a study by *Libow* (1974). All of these studies represent attempts to define physiological, psychological and social predictors of longevity which effect survival in old age. *Rose and Bell* (1971) offered a model which tries to integrate information on the interrelationships between these groups of predictors while placing special emphasis on the role of social factors (fig. 1).

Several of the more recent studies, including the Bonn Longitudinal Study of Aging (BLSA), have contributed to a more differentiated view of these interrelationships. Although there exist some differences between these studies re-

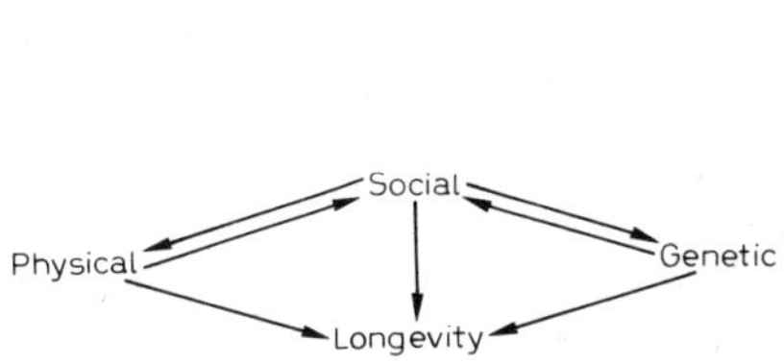

Fig. 1. Interrelationships among social, physical and genetic influences on longevity (from *Rose and Bell,* 1971, p. 20).

garding the role attributed to each of these variables for survivorship, nobody denies the complexity and interdependency of the conditions of survival. This common core of findings points to the great methodological problems connected with our topic and raises some doubts about the validity of results of several well-known studies on centenarians. This is especially true for studies which approach the problem of longevity with highly developed batteries of biological and clinical tests, while relying on very naive forms of interviews of intuitive interpretation of expressive movements for the study of psychological and social aspects of the problem.

One line of research on the causes of longevity addressed itself to the analysis of *statistical material* available for large populations. Another methodological approach to the task of finding out what leads to long life is the systematic scientific study of *aged individuals*. Examples of this type of study can be seen in the work of *Franke* (1971a, b, 1973), *Franke and Schmitt* (1971), *Franke et al.* (1970, 1973) in Germany, *Haranghy et al.* (1965) in Hungary, *Lambrev* (1951) in Bulgaria, and *Chebotarev* (1969) in the USSR. The groundwork for the most important type of inquiry was laid by the challenge confronting every *longitudinal study* to analyze its sample reduction in as much detail as possible, since the shrunken sample might not have remained comparable to the original sample. The attempt was made to carry out thorough analyses of dropouts, that is, cases for which no data were available in subsequent testing sessions. Not all dropouts resulted from deaths, of course, and comparisons were carried out for medical, sociological, and psychological data from the initial testing.

In the present context, however, interest is focused on the group for whom continued participation was made impossible by death. Extensive information has been presented by *Riegel* (1969) using material from a gerontological study he initiated in 1956/57 in northern Germany. He attempted to gather new information from the same 380 subjects 5 years later in 1961/62. First session scores were used to compare the group who died before the first follow-up session and with those who participated in the second follow-up testing. This comparison revealed correlations of longevity with higher verbal scores on the Hamburg-Wechsler intelligence test (German standardization of the WAIS), as well as with a more widely differentiated range of interests and lower rigidity and dogmatism scores. This finding is supported by *Libow* (1974), who compared the survivors and nonsurvivors of the Bethesda Study of Aging (*Birren et al.,* 1963b) on the basis of data from the first measurement point. The data from the Veterans Administration Study (*Rose and Bell,* 1971) do not offer a very clear picture concerning differences between survivors and nonsurvivors. These differences change from cohort to cohort. Generally, physical factors seem to be more predictive for survivorship than psychological or social variables (*Richardson,* 1973; *Mueller et al.,* 1975). Still another combination of predictors for longevity was found in an analysis of the Duke Longitudinal Study of Aging which was done by *Pfeiffer* (1969). It pointed to remarkable sex differences in the relevance of predictors for longevity. For women, most of the variance was explained by IQ, perceived change in health status, and family status, whereas, for men, socioeconomic status, perceived change in health status, and physiological status were more decisive.

In conclusion, we can refer to *Pfeiffer* (1974, p. 28) who states in his summary of longitudinal findings on the correlates of 'survival' that there appears to be no single factor which determines longevity but rather a constellation of biological, psychological, and social factors, amounting to what may best be described as elite status. In the light of these findings, the BLSA can be expected to add only some new nuances to the definition of factors which, as a total constellation, are correlated with survivorship.

BLSA Findings

Survivor and Nonsurvivor Samples

Of the 222 men and women comprising the BLSA sample at the first measurement point in 1965, 45 were no longer alive at the last measurement point in 1972, and 57% declined to take part in the last session due to their own personal illness or that of a member of the family. Deaths between the first and fifth measurement points constituted 18.2% of the women and 22% of the men in the original sample. As expected, the older cohort (1890–1895) had a higher percentage of death, 28%, than the younger cohort (1900–1905) with 13.5%.

Results

Biological Correlates of Survival

At the first measurement point, nonsurvivors had more sclerotic symptoms and lower auditive capacity than survivors. There was no difference, however, in respect to physician's rating of general health, cardiovascular insufficiency, vision, and the degree of physical mobility during the last year (table I). In interviews conducted as part of the testing, survivors expressed more concern about their health than did nonsurvivors. An analysis of variance with the factors sex and survivorship confirmed the difference in auditive capacity between the two groups, especially among the men. Further results of this analysis revealed that in the year preceding the first measurement period, the nonsurvivors had consulted their doctors significantly less often than the survivors (table I).

Cognitive Functioning

WAIS (HAWIE) data from the BLSA revealed the same striking difference between intelligence scores of survivors and nonsurvivors previously reported in

Table I. Means and standard deviations of medical data from survivors and nonsurvivors

	Survivors			*Nonsurvivors*		
	number	mean	SD	number	mean	SD
General health status	117	2.0	0.9	39	2.9	0.8
Sclerotic symptoms	114	1.2	0.8	37	1.1	0.8
Caediobascular insufficiency	116	1.3	0.6	38	1.3	0.5
Vision	117	1.9	1.0	38	1.8	0.9
Hearing	117	1.8	1.0	38	1.5	0.9
Degree of physical mobility	115	1.2	0.5	38	1.1	0.4

Table II. Means and standard deviations of intelligence scores of survivors and nonsurvivors

	Survivor			Nonsurvivor		
	number	mean	SD	number	mean	SD
General information	119	10.7	2.5	40	9.5	2.9
General comprehension	119	11.9	2.2	40	10.6	2.9
Arithmetic	119	9.6	2.5	40	8.8	2.0
Similarities	119	9.7	2.2	40	9.2	2.5
Vocabulary (digit span)	119	10.5	2.3	40	9.5	3.1
Picture completion	119	7.4	2.2	40	6.1	2.3
Picture arrangement	119	8.7	2.5	40	7.7	2.7
Block design	119	9.1	3.0	40	7.8	3.6
Object assembly	119	8.8	2.5	40	7.1	2.9
Coding (mazes)	119	9.5	2.9	40	8.7	3.4
Verbal scores	119	52.4	8.8	40	47.5	11.4
Performance scores	119	43.4	9.5	40	36.7	12.1
Total scores	119	95.8	17.0	40	84.2	22.1

other longitudinal studies. This difference pertains to the total IQ as well as to the portion and, particularly, the performance scores where a difference of 6.7 points was found. In the analysis of variance for all data, the strongest contrasts between survivors and nonsurvivors occurred in the verbal scores and figure and numerical reasoning. The group effect for the total scores disappeared in the analysis of variance (table II and III).

Table III. HAWIE subtest means for the significant and very significant effects of the analyses of variance

	Male	Female	Survivor	Nonsurvivor
General information	11.5	9.5	10.7	10.9
General comprehension	12.3	10.7	11.3	11.9
Arithmetic	9.9	8.5	9.6	8.7
Similarities	10.9	9.5	10.5	10.0
Picture comprehension	9.1	8.3	8.7	7.7
Picture arrangement	9.8	7.5	9.1	8.5
Block design	8.4	8.1	8.8	7.8
Object assembly	9.5	8.7	9.4	7.8
Verbal scores	53.8	47.4	52.3	48.9
Performance scores	43.1	38.4	43.2	38.3
Total scores	96.2	85.7	95.4	86.6

Table IV. Means and standard deviations for psychomotor performance (Mierke apparatus) and Riegel attitude scales

	Survivors			Nunsurvivors		
	number	mean	SD	number	mean	SD
Miercke 50%	106	198.0	35.7	33	206.4	44.8
Riegel scales						
AR	115	17.8	4.1	38	19.2	4.6
PR	115	14.7	4.7	38	16.0	4.5
IN	115	5.0	3.3	38	4.8	3.0
AD	115	17.3	3.5	38	16.6	4.4
L_6	115	14.7	4.6	38	13.5	4.2
L_7	115	14.4	3.6	38	14.1	3.4

Psychomotor Performance

Psychomotor performance on the Mierke apparatus (*Mathey,* 1975) should be a good predictor of survival, since it is closely related to high speed information processing. The analysis of variance confirms this expectation by demonstrating that the survivors reached the 50-percent correct response criterion faster (average 198) than the nonsurvivors (average 206.4; table IV).

Cognitive Style and Attitudes

The four Riegel scales supposed to measure different aspects of rigidity – general rigidity (AR), personal rigidity (PR), intolerance (IN), and general dogmatism (AD) – may be regarded as indicators of a cognitive style. The expectation that rigidity as a typical reaction to stress should be higher in nonsurvivors was not supported by our data. Differences in the scores for general rigidity and personal rigidity, however, did point in the anticipated direction. Scores on scales measuring attitude toward past or future (L_6) and attitude toward the present (L_7) did not differentiate between the two groups.

Personality Ratings

Additional information on personality was available in the form of ratings. The expectation that these ratings would differentiate between survivors and nonsurvivors was supported by the results of an analysis of variance, especially the ratings of activity and adjustment. At the first measurement point, the survivors were also marked by their better mood or morale. These results are illustrated by table V.

Social Correlates of Survivorship

Information on social participation was gathered by means of interview schedules and rating scales based on those from the cross-national study of adjustment to retirment (*Havighurst et al.*, 1969). Survivors and nonsurvivors did not differ significantly in terms of social participation at the first point of measurement. An analysis of variance identified only one point over which the groups expressed different role satisfaction, namely satisfaction with the role of neighbor. However, survivors reported that they felt needed to a significantly higher proportion than nonsurvivors. Tables VI and VII provide more detailed findings on social variables.

Table V. Means and standard deviations of personality ratings

	Survivors			Nonsurvivors		
	number	mean	SD	number	mean	SD
Activity	120	6.2	1.2	40	5.4	1.3
Changes in activity	120	4.4	1.2	40	4.3	1.2
Form of activity	120	5.8	1.4	40	5.1	1.7
Mood	120	5.6	1.3	40	5.0	1.3
Changes in mood	120	4.6	1.3	40	4.5	1.4
Responsiveness	120	6.2	1.2	40	5.7	1.7
Adjustment	120	5.8	1.3	40	5.9	1.4
Self-control	120	5.4	1.0	40	5.3	1.3
Security	120	5.5	1.2	40	5.1	1.2

Table VI. Means and standard deviations for activity in various social roles

Role	Survivors			Nonsurvivors		
	number	mean	SD	number	mean	SD
Parent	105	6.2	2.1	26	6.1	2.3
Grandparent	115	4.9	1.4	40	4.3	1.7
Relative	72	1.8	2.1	26	1.5	1.4
Friend	100	3.0	2.3	35	3.5	2.1
Acquaintance	116	3.1	1.6	39	3.0	1.5
Neighbor	117	7.2	2.2	39	7.1	2.4
Club member	109	5.1	1.9	32	5.4	2.0
Spouse	111	5.9	3.0	37	6.1	3.4
Citizen	102	2.9	1.7	40	2.7	1.4

Table VII. Means and standard deviations in degree of satisfaction with various roles

	Survivors			Nonsurvivors		
	number	mean	SD	number	mean	SD
Satisfaction with parent role	113	7.1	1.9	39	6.7	2.5
Satisfaction with grandparent role	86	5.2	2.8	23	5.6	2.3
Satisfaction with relative role	107	3.8	1.9	36	4.0	1.9
Satisfaction with friend role	100	2.9	2.3	33	3.5	2.2
Satisfaction with acquaintance role	119	4.2	2.8	40	4.2	3.1
Satisfaction with neighbor role	115	4.4	3.1	38	4.1	3.1
Satisfaction with club mumber role	120	3.0	1.4	40	3.1	1.4
Satisfaction with spouse role	117	6.1	2.9	40	6.6	2.8
Satisfaction with citizen role	112	6.9	2.0	36	7.0	2.0
Feeling needed	112	7.8	2.1	38	6.5	2.6

Table VIII. Means and standard deviations for leisure activities

Activity	Survivors			Nonsurvivors		
	number	mean	SD	number	mean	SD
Newspaper reading	115	1.6	1.2	40	1.7	1.3
Travel	120	6.0	2.4	40	5.8	2.6
Gardening	118	2.2	0.9	40	2.1	0.9
Being visited	120	3.0	2.8	40	3.0	2.7
Paying visits	120	5.3	2.1	40	5.8	2.7
Entertainment with others	120	4.6	1.9	40	5.5	2.4
Going to the movies	36	2.0	1.2	40	2.4	1.1
Going out for something to eat or drink	117	3.6	2.8	39	3.1	2.2
Attending church	113	1.5	1.6	38	1.3	1.2
Going for a walk	31	1.3	1.3	12	1.2	1.4
Taking an excursion	27	1.7	1.5	14	1.5	1.4
Reading magazines	102	2.9	1.8	37	2.4	1.8
Listening to the radio	111	4.3	2.0	39	4.3	1.9
Television viewing	117	3.6	2.4	40	2.5	1.7

Leisure Activity

Reports on leisure activities at the first measurement point did not reveal any significant differences between survivors and nonsurvivors. Differences obtained by analyses of variance were linked to uninterpretable effects, e. g. reading magazines, television viewing, and going out for something to eat or drink (table VIII).

Perceived Life Situation and Survivorship

Survivors tended toward higher satisfaction and a more positive outlook toward the future, but there were no significant differences between survivors and nonsurvivors in the actual variables such as perceived housing stress, housing conditions, family situation, or physical impairment. Both survivors and nonsurvivors rated their average day as fairly unchanging.

Summary and Discussion

The BLSA findings on correlates of survivorship in longitudinal studies generally correspond to those of previous studies (*Pfeiffer,* 1969). Contrary to findings by *Rose and Bell* (1971), *Richardson* (1973), and *Mueller et al.* (1975), no definite health differences were found between survivors and nonsurvivors. This may be due to the procedure by which medical data were gathered and to our sampling procedures, which favored the selection of healthy persons. On the other hand, we are in agreement with those writers who found decisive differences between survivors and nonsurvivors in terms of IQ and personality variables such as activity and mood.

Our survivors did not differ from nonsurvivors regarding social activity and satisfaction with degree of activity. However, more survivors felt needed than nonsurvivors. No major differences were found between the two groups in regard to family, job, and economic situation. The correlation between IQ and survivorship, which has become evident in a number of studies, needs further clarification. It was not confirmed for women in studies like that of *Britton and Britton* (1969). As far as studies on women are available at all, they point to the interaction between sex, intelligence, and socioeconomic status. Although socioeconomic status and IQ correlate very highly with survivorship in men, this is not true for women, because their socioeconomic status is often defined in relevant studies by their husband's socioeconomic status. Taking the contradictory findings on the correlations between socioeconomic status and IQ for men and women into consideration, we may conclude that, in the BLSA age cohort, survivorship correlates with socioeconomic status more than with age or other variables. There are, of course, also other factors of relevance to survivorship.

A major finding of our study and other studies concerns the importance of personality variables like activity, morale, and adjustment, all of which facilitate active coping behavior. The effect of these variables, however, is not restricted to certain social classes.

Greater activity provides both sensory and social stimulation, widens the range of interests, and opens the opportunity for more contact with other people. As far as we can tell, data from this and other studies support the conclusion that such activity stimulates cognitive activities.

Apparently, we are dealing here with a process of interactions. Aged persons who are more active show more initiative in various areas of life. They are more involved, more open-minded, and more interested in their physical and social surroundings. At the same time, cognitive functioning benefits from this stimulation and 'training'. A further characteristic of activity deserves mention in this context. More than IQ or socioeconomic status, activity is correlated with how the aged persons in our study coped with crisis situations such as illness, physical stress, or emotional stress. An integrative model of those findings is graphically illustrated by figure 2. This model shows that genetic (1) and ecological factors (2) not only combine to affect longevity directly, but also influence intelligence (3) and personality, including activity (4).

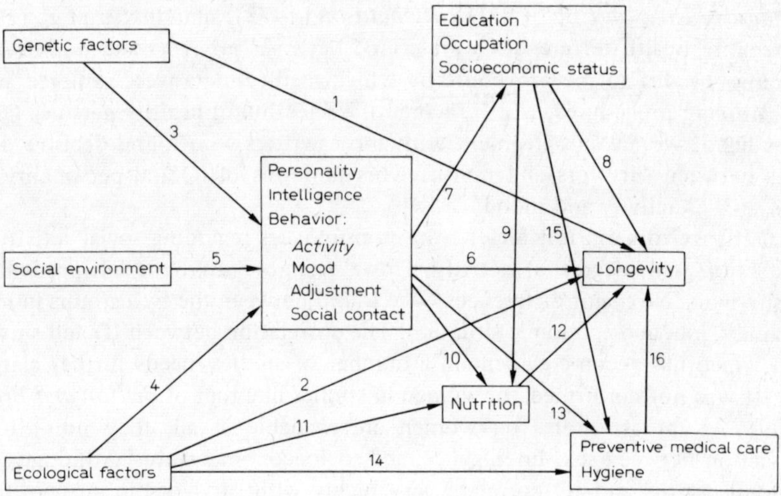

Fig. 2. Determinants of longevity.

Intelligence and personality, in turn, are also determined to a large extent by the social environment (5), for example by parental child-raising practices, etc. The effects of personality and intelligence take different forms. They appear to have both a direct influence on longevity (6), and an indirect influence in terms of their connection (at least for men) with better education (7) and higher socioeconomic status, which both (8) are identifiable as direct correlates of longevity. Better education not only augments personality, intelligence, and certain environmental conditions, but also serves as a prerequisite for more qualified occupations, which once again lead to longevity via improved socioeconomic status. Social status (9), coupled with a particular personality (10) and other environmental conditions (11) ensures proper nutrition, which is a further correlate of longevity (12). Similarly, personality (13), ecological conditions (14), socioeconomic status (15) and nutrition go hand in hand with preventive medical care and attention to hygiene (16).

This model still may not include all relevant variables. In any case it demonstrates the highly complex interaction between 'external' and 'internal', social, physiological, and psychological conditions of longevity. More research is necessary to study the complicated interaction between these and other variables. Above all, studies designed to take account of all the measures identifiable as relevant at our present state of knowledge and study them using multivariate statistical methods hold promise.

Contr. hum. Dev., vol. 3, pp. 147–161 (Karger, Basel 1976)

XII. Patterns of „Succesful" Aging

Conclusions from the Bonn Longitudinal Study of Aging

H. Thomae

'Normal' Aging and 'Successful' Aging

In his introduction to the first summarizing report on the Duke Longitudinal Study on Aging, *Palmore* (1970, p. VI) defined this study as one dealing with 'normal aging' in terms of 'non-institutionalized' aging and aging rather free from 'unusual abnormalities'. The same is true for the population of our study. The publications on our previous findings have contributed and will contribute to a major revision of the prevailing image of aging in Western Europe (*Thomae,* 1968a–d; *Lehr,* 1971a, b). This negative stereotype of aging very often is oriented on the small percentage of institutionalized persons (in the Federal Republic of Germany in 1971: 2.26%) and even more on experiences with physically or mentally handicapped aged patients. Therefore, we also might have designated our study as one on 'normal aging', especially as most of our findings are in agreement with those of the Duke and similar longitudinal studies.

We might therefore have summarized a great deal of our findings by quoting Palmore's *(1970) statements on the high degree of consistency of cognitive functioning, activities and attitudes in old age (pp. 420–422). For our subjects we would have to make some additional statements, however, pointing to a high degree of stability in personality variables like activity, adjustment, mood (morale), ego control and emotional stability.* In this respect, our longitudinal sample, although less biased in terms of socioeconomic status (SES) than the Duke Study, might be considered even more an 'elite group physically, mentally, and socially' (*Palmore,* 1970, p. 422) than the Duke Study.

From our findings we cannot support the finding of *Busse et al.,* (1970) according to which the majority of an aged sample like the Duke 'elite group' showed psychoneurotic, mixed, organic or even psychotic symptoms. Perhaps this finding could not be confirmed in the follow-up study, as it is not mentioned in the second publication (*Palmore,* 1974a, b). In our sample there was one subject with a psychotic background who died in a mental hospital. The others showed a rather normal distribution of adjustment, mood and emotional responsiveness. Apparently it is mostly a matter of convenience how we classify cases below or above the median of rating scales for these personality aspects. We can call them 'psychoneurotic' or 'low in adjustment', we can designate them as cases with 'depressive' reactions or as 'low in mood'. In the first case we have labeled them as psychiatric cases although they never need psychiatric help. In the latter case we deal with them as normal persons, just like their families, their friends, or neighbors. As a matter of fact, if we would apply the 'diagnostic instrument' of *Busse et al.* (1970) and other psychiatrists to the study of persons in young and middle adulthood, we would get the same distribution of psychiatric symptoms as in the old group, provided that we were able to do this rating without bias, i. e. without knowledge of the age of the panel.

Considering the high degree of 'normality' and of continuously well-adjusted behavior in the survivors of longitudinal studies, one might define the aging process of such a group as an example of 'successful aging'. By doing so we would avoid the problem of delineating the degree of 'normality' in terms of 'averageness' of this group. Perhaps this 'normal' or 'average' process of aging can be found in an area between the 'elite' life of our survivors on the one hand and that of less successful, ill, and/or disabled persons living in institutions on the other hand. It will not be easy to rate the distance between this 'successful' group and the area of 'normal aging'. However, this normal area is to be located closer to the successful pattern than to the patterns defined by increase of dependency, helplessness, or social isolation.

According to findings with a random cross-sectional sample covering the age range 65–90, we can locate the 'normal' group rather close to the 'elite' group of the BLSA survivors (*Schmitz-Scherzer et al.,* 1974). This sample (415 men and women, age 65–80) was studied from a medical, sociological, and psychological point of view at Münster, Westphalia. It will be referred to, therefore, as the Münster sample. The Münster sample medians for cognitive functioning, psychomotor performance, and personality variables like activity were only 0.2–1.5 points below those of our longitudinal sample. Another difference between this cross-sectional sample and the BLSA sample refers to social isolation. Whereas most of our subjects reported a high degree of social participation (chap. IX, p. xxx), there was a greater percentage of perceived isolation in the Münster sample (*Schmitz-Scherzer et al.,* 1974): 18.8% of the men and 29% of the women said that 'isolation' was the greatest problem in their life. Another area of concern was income: 15.1% of the men and 11.8% of the women reported serious problems in this area compared to 5–7% who did so in the BLSA. Finally, there was a difference regarding health: while this was rated as 'average' to 'good' in BLSA by the physician, 50% of the Münster sample suffered from at least two health problems (especially coronary and respiratory diseases and orthopedic problems).

As the social stratification of the BLSA and the Münster sample were identical, we might hypothesize that the differences in cognitive functioning, social participation and perceived economic situation are to be explained primarily by different coping techniques. Perhaps the better health of the BLSA sample enabled our subjects to respond to their problems in the active manner which according to *Lehr and Schmitz-Scherzer* (chap. XI, p. xxx) is a main correlate of survivorship.

Generally, however, a cross-sectional sample of non-institutionalized aged persons is very similar to our longitudinal sample and very much unlike a sample of institutionalized and mentally or physically disabled persons. Therefore, successful aging defined by survivorship in our sample comes rather close to 'normal aging', and if there exists something like 'elite' aging (like that of 'centenarian' or 'professional' persons), it will be still a different pattern of aging, not that of the BLSA subjects.

Criteria for the Classification of Patterns of Aging

It would simplify our problem if we would solve the task of a differential gerontology by classifying aged persons into the three or four groups defined so far ('elite', survivorship in the BLSA, 'normal aging' like in the Münster sample, 'institutionalized and/or impaired' aging.) Obviously there can be a great degree of 'normality' regarding personality variables like 'ego control' or 'emotional responsiveness' even in institutionalized groups. Therefore, the three or four patterns defined so far are cues for a general orientation which should be used in any statement on the 'aging process'. Statements of this kind are misleading if they are oriented toward the extreme patterns (centenarians versus chronically ill, poor, or disabled aged), however, the distorting effect of the 'extreme' orientation will be less dangerous if 'survivors' in longitudinal studies are used as models for the definition of 'aging' compared to a clinical orientation which uses deterioration as the 'normal' case.

Differential gerontology will define many patterns between normal and elite aging, between normal and abnormal or pathological aging. These definitions will also vary, due to the many possible criteria for differentiation. Life-styles as defined by *Havighurst et al.* (1964), *Havighurst and de Vries* (1969) and *Maas and Kuypers* (1974) are variations of social participation or performance of social roles in the aged. *Reichard et al.* (1962) used attitudinal variables for their descriptions of different forms of aging.

Havighurst (1975) combined the classifications of *Reichard et al.* (1962) on the one hand and those of his co-workers ending up with eight personality types in old age like, e. g., (1) re-organizers: 'competent people engaged in a wide variety of activity'; (2) integrated-focused: 'they tend to be selective in their activities and gain satisfaction from this concentration on one or two roles', and (8) disorganized: 'they have deteriorated thought processes and poor control over their emotions'. *Havighurst* (1975) assumes that these patterns 'are established and predictable by middle age'. This shows that he believes that 'patterns of aging' are rather consequences of individual choices than outcomes of social, biological, and biographical constellations.

On the other hand, as 'aging' can be defined as a series of events the individual has to cope with, 'patterns' of aging can be defined in terms of the degree and the ways in which a balance between the individual and social system is attained. This is the main point of view in the approach to life-styles as defined by *Williams and Wirths* (1965). They assert that an autonomy-dependency dimension defines the degree and the manner of attaining or restoring the balance between person and social system. An autonomous person is a person in balance or one who is maintaining a balance by more energy output. A dependent person requires more input from others to maintain a balance. We shall refer to this classification in suggesting different strategies in problem solving as a most relevant classification of patterns of aging.

Another source of unbalance is defined by awareness of death. *Munnichs* (1966) found five major variants of attitudes toward death: 'ignoring', 'escape', 'evasion', 'acquiescence', and 'acceptance' and demonstrated how they are combined with certain global patterns of conditions and behaviors in old age.

Finally we should mention that certain 'patterns' of aging are derived also from ideas which critisize the overestimation of IQ measures in the assessment of the aged. *Fisher* (1973) suggested replacing the assessment of elderly persons via IQ measures by measures of cognitive and social accessibility. These two dimensions are supplemented by a third defined as being likeable. These three dimensions would define a great number of 'aging patterns' in terms of behavioral tendencies which are immediately relevant for the life situation of the aged.

'Patterns' of Successful Aging as Defined by Longitudinal Data

The foregoing chapters of this volume pointed to several variables which are correlated with each other consistently through the period of observation (i. e. from measurement point, MP, I–V). From these consistent clusters we might conclude that poor SES, poor health, poor cognitive functioning, lower degree of social activity, and lower morale form a pattern which differs distinctly from an opposite form, defined by consistently better SES, health, cognitive functioning, and better personality adjustment.

However, the chapters of this book dealing with different behavioral aspects demonstrate that the patterns defined by SES, health, IQ, social participation, and general adjustment are more 'ideal types' than 'real' groups. Firstly, there are effects of cohort and sex which can compensate or reinforce the effects of SES or health. On the other hand, the composition of these patterns may change to a certain degree in different behavioral aspects. Whereas SES was consistently correlated to cognitive functioning (chap. III, p. xxx), there was no consistent correlation regarding health. In the multiple choice reaction test there existed a consistent correlation between health and performance. The differences in the performance of different occupational groups were reversed in women compared to men: only in this women group, former white-collar employees showed better performance in this test. In the simple reaction task devised by *Beck, Mathey* (chap. IV, p. 47) did not find any correlations between test performance and health or personality.

Regarding personality as measured by L data (rating scales) *Grombach* (chap. V, p. 61) points to a consistent correlation between social status and consistency and change of behavioral tendencies. However, this correlation is related to different aspects of behavior in men and women. 'Ego control' is more related to social status in men, 'activity' and 'responsiveness' more in women. Obviously 'ego control' belongs to the main characteristics of the female role, at least for the cohorts concerned, whereas high 'activity', and responsiveness are related more to middle-class status than to lower status in women.

There are other examples for sex- or cohort-specific correlations between social, health, and psychological variables as studied in a longitudinal sample. Health accounted rather constantly for about 10% of the variance over time regarding 'adjustment' in men, whereas this proportion of variance dropped to 0.2% in women (chap. V, p. 62). We might relate this finding again to aspects of the female role as defined for these cohorts. 'Adjustment' to the requirements of a 1-week psychological testing program included more definite norms independent of health for women than for men.

Regarding 'rigidity' as measured by the Riegel scales, SES turned out to be the main determinant for the classification of 'low' versus 'high' scores at each of the points of measurement (chap. VI, p. 74). However, this finding could not be replicated when verbal intelligence was controlled. Therefore, it would be misleading to correlate SES directly with rigidity in attitudes.

Olbrich and Lehr (chap. IX, p. 124) point to the problems involved in a 'global' assessment of consistency and change in social participation. Whereas psychological variables like feeling of well-being and other measures of life space were not related to changes in family roles over time, they were related to changes in extrafamilial roles.. SES did not function as a major principle for the definition of consistency and change in social participation.

From the study of patterns of consistency and change in leisure behavior *Schmitz-Scherzer* (chap. X, p. 129) concludes that a great amount of individual variation may be related to SES, health, and personality. However, he believes that changes in the personal situation of the individual may be related even more to the frequent changes of activities as observed during the observation period. Generally, he would doubt if the definition of 'patterns of aging' in terms of leisure activity will be possible from a longitudinal point of view.

On the other hand, *Fisseni* (chap. VIII, p. 96) demonstrated by use of configuration frequential analyses how patterns of aging can be derived from interview data related to different aspects of the life space. These longitudinal patterns are very often sex- and/or cohort-specific and point to influences of health as well as SES. Their great variety demonstrates the variety of behavioral sequences of developmental processes which occur in the process of redefining an individual life space again and again as this is made necessary by changes in the physical, social, and psychological situation of the aged.

From all this evidence, the view of aging emerging in these papers demonstrates that the pattern of successful aging, as defined by survivorship (versus nonsurvivorship) in chapter XI (p. 137), is only a global description. It actually provides information on the conditions for aging in the survivor group at the beginning of the study.

The sequence of external events or of changes or maintained consistencies in behavior which started at MPI can apparently be explained by a very complex interaction of processes. Due to this complexity (this chap. p. 161), *Schmitz-Scherzer* (1975b) and *Thomae* (1968a-c) wonder if it will be necessary to turn to the study of single cases, the number of our subjects being too small for a statistical analysis of combinations of variables in a longitudinal way. By doing so, *Mathey* (chap. IV, p. 46) found that psychomotor performance measured by the Mierke apparatus was consistently higher in those persons who showed above-average cognitive functioning, who consistently reported positive expectations for the future, and whose life conditions included a 'moderate' degree of stress in economic, housing, and family matters, etc. If perceived stress was high, it had adverse effects. This pattern certainly corresponds to that of 'active coping' which is the focus of the pattern correlated to 'survivorship' or longevity (chap. XI, p. 145).

Schmitz-Scherzer (1975a, b) concludes from his methodological evaluation of the BLSA data that the variety of 'patterns' of consistency and change, which became evident in the pool of longitudinal data, will resist any systematic classification.

Styles of Successful Aging and Cognitive Theory of Aging

Although there exist strong tendencies in contemporary psychology toward a renaissance of the study of single cases – promoted e. g. by studies on behavior therapies, biofeedback, and similar techniques – the authors of this volume feel that there are some alternatives to this method. Some of us will test some new statistical techniques – like path analysis – in order to derive patterns from our data pool. Others will wait for the next follow-up study, since the 7- to 8-year span between MP I and MP V may not be long enough.

Still another alternative is the concentration on a set of variables which are especially relevant for the prediction of behavior. Our study confirmed the finding of many writers according to whom cognitive variables like perceived stress, perceived degree of social participation, perceived health, or income very often are more correlated to consistency and change in behavior than objective measures of social conditions (chap. IV, p. 46, chap. V, p. 65 and chap IX, p. 124; *Opgenoorth,* 1971; *Schreiner,* 1969; *Theissen,* 1970a, b; *Tismer,* 1971). These findings are in agreement with cognitive theories of behavior, according to which the 'cognitive representation of the situation' is the 'effective environment' for the organism (*Baldwin,* 1969). In a previous paper (*Thomae,* 1970) we quoted clinical observations according to which a fatal illness like cancer will not influence the well-being and adjustment of a person unless he is feeling pain or is being told the 'truth'.

Another argument for the first postulate of the 'cognitive theory of aging' (*Thomae,* 1970) is offered by studies on correlates of adjustment to retirement. The way retirement was perceived and anticipated is one of the best predictors for successful adjustment (*Ash,* 1966; *Lehr and Dreher,* 1969). The same is true for adjustment to institutionalization. *Lieberman et al.* (1968) as well as *Lehr* (1970) demonstrated that the way institutionalization was anticipated is more closely related to the adjustment, morale and time perspective of institutionalized people than the conditions in the institutions themselves.

Further evidence for a cognitive theory of aging is provided by studies on antecedents of suicide in old age. *Wiendieck* (1973) found that serious suicidal intentions were correlated to the 'subjective evaluation' of the person's own situation and to negative expectancies for the future rather than to the objective situation as defined by illness, social isolation, loss of spouse, or retirement.

We might define many patterns of aging in terms of the major dimensions of cognitive representation of the situation. *Schreiner* (1969, 1971) analyzed relationships between extension and quality of future time perspective on the one hand and social and biological background as well as behavioral variables on the other hand. *Theissen* (1970a, b) analyzed different informations on self-concept among our subjects and found the same complex interrelationships between different qualities of self-concept and behavioral as well as social variables.

Other findings from BLSA supporting this hypothesis which could not be included in this book are related to perceived versus objective health and behavior (*Lehr et al.,* 1972) or to problems of intergenerational conflict. *Merker* (1973) concluded from her findings in analyses of our data concerning attitude to the younger generation that this most relevant behavioral aspect was more closely related to perceived life space (others and self) than to 'objective' (i. e. stimulus-defined) conditions of life.

A very complex interaction between variables of perceived life space and behavioral variables was demonstrated also in research on 'life satisfaction' as the 'cognitive representation' of adjustment to aging (*Havighurst,* 1963) or attained social competence (*Kuypers and Bengston,* 1973). According to *Adams* (1973), research on correlates of life satisfaction identified 50–70 variables which include socioeconomic, social, health and psychological variables. The psychological variables included in this list referred entirely to other 'cognitive' constructs. As any of these conditions may change due to own or other's illness or impairment or due to loss of 'significant others', it can be expected that the degree of satisfaction is more like a 'level of adaptation' (*Helson,* 1964) fluctuating around a standard which may be raised or lowered according to external or internal conditions.

This may be expected, too, by postulate II of the 'cognitive theory of aging', according to which any change in the situation is perceived and evaluated in terms of the dominant concerns and expectations of the individual (*Thomae,* 1970, p. 5). This postulate introduces motivational aspects as intervening between change of situation and perception of this change. Due to the intervening function of motivational variables, attitudes, etc., loss of some roles (e.g. neighbor or relative) may not be perceived as a major change whereas a moderate drop in contacts with children or grandchildren may result in the belief that 'my whole life has been changed'.

We shall have to analyze our data in terms of these motivational states, in order to be able to correlate our data on measured consistency and change in behavior to measured change in the 'objective', social, economic, housing, or health status. Anyhow, the definition of 'patterns of aging' in terms of dimensions of 'life space' and of 'self-concept' will add some meaningful information to knowledge on the differentiating consequences of health, social status and background as well as role performance, as demonstrated in this book.

Another set of 'patterns' may be deduced from postulate III of the 'cognitive theory of aging', according to which 'adjustment to aging is a function of the balance between cognitive and motivational systems of the individual' (*Thomae,* 1970, p. 8). This postulate is based on the close correlation between 'life satisfaction' as a general measure of 'adjustment' on the one hand (*Havighurst,* 1963) and 'cognitive representations of the situation' (*Baldwin,* 1969) on the other hand (*Adams,* 1973).

These correlations are misleading, however, if they are interpreted in terms of a 'solid', 'consistent' cognitive structure and a solid, unchanging quality of life satisfaction. From our longitudinal observations we would expect a high degree of fluctuation in these 'cognitive representations' (such as self-concept, future time perspective, satisfaction with family or occupational role) and, consequently, a fluctuation of 'life satisfaction'. Therefore, any study on adjustment in aging which does not define how this balance between motivational and cognitive balance is restored again and again will miss some of the most relevant aspects of aging. On the basis of ample information we might define the 'focal developmental task of old age' (*Havighurst,* 1972) in terms of the maintenance of a minimum of 'affective balance' (*Moriwak,* 1974), 'life satisfaction', or 'social competence' (*Kuypers and Bengston,* 1973) in a situation which is bound to be unbalanced for biological, psychological, and social reasons. This evaluation of the situation of aged people should not be confounded with 'deficit models' of aging which cannot be supported by our findings on cognitive functioning and general adjustment. The annual or biennial reports of our subjects on their life situations did include many indications of disturbed balance which could, however, be restored by external as well as internal activities.

This is also shown in studies on situation-specific changes in the self-concept of aged persons (*Theissen,* 1970a, b; *Peters,* 1971). *Eisdorfer* (1968) concludes from careful studies that motivational variables like anxiety interfere with cognitive functioning in aging. As this interference is explained by the hypothesis of a higher (instead of a lower) arousal level in the aged, one might doubt if this argument can be used as an indicator of situation-specific regulations. On the other hand, we recognize the fairly good social adjustment of aged persons who score low in cognitive tasks. Therefore, the interference of 'high arousal' and performance can be regarded as situation-specific.

A stressful character is attributed to the aging process *per se* by *Rosow* (1973). Although this view overemphasizes some of the existing problems, the data given by *Rosow* certainly point to the continuous exposure of the aged to problems which have to be coped with and which may result in an increased arousal level with many situation-specific fluctuations.

Considering these evaluations of the situation confronting many elderly persons, we can define the genuine task of life in old age as the continuous restoration of emotional, and/or behavioral balance in a situation of increased potential for imbalance.

Patterns of Aging as Strategies in Problem Solving

If this is true, the definition of 'patterns' of aging should be oriented toward this most relevant aspect of human life in old age. 'Patterns of aging' from this point of view are different forms of restoration of this balance (*Williams and Wirths,* 1965). The set of variables measured in our research program also includes assessments of these 'problem-solving processes'. They have not been dealt with in a separate chapter because the analysis of these data will require refined rating procedures and statistical techniques. Some of the previous publications (*Thomae and Simons,* 1967; *Langermann-Erlenkamp,* 1970) and some unpublished studies, however, enable us to report how the problem of defining 'patterns of aging' in a psychologically relevant way might be solved in the near future.

As mentioned before (p. xxx), one of the interviews included in the study concentrated on the socioeconomic, occupational, family, and housing situation as it existed for the person at the time of the currency reform in 1948. As most of the respondents had to face many problems at that time, there existed fairly good chances that the interview would elicit memories of the problems themselves and how they were dealt with. Therefore we took information on problem situations existing immediately after the war and patterns of adjustment to these situations as the basis for the classification of these adjustment patterns. First we got a list of approximately 25 such patterns which then had to be reduced to 15, since in the reference times 1955 and 1965 most of them did not exist anymore.

These adjustment patterns were rated on 9-point scales by trained raters. Conference ratings as well as control ratings by two to five raters were made, resulting in a 85-percent inter-rater agreement. The rank order of adjustment patterns in the reports of men (born 1900–1905) on the area of occupational problems in 1948 and 1965 is given in table I (according to *Thomae and Simons,* 1967).

The rank order correlation between the adjustment patterns reported for 1948 and 1965 is not significant. The difference in the structure of overall adjustment to the situation is explained especially by differences in the rating scores for four adjustment patterns. 'Adjustment to the institutional aspects of the situation', i.e. adjustment by applying to the employment office, the former employer, the trade union, or local authorities was most important for getting or keeping a job in 1948. It was not so important in 1965 when half of these men were retired and problems in this area usually had to do with getting the highest possible pension or finding a postretirement job.

Another major 'technique' or 'adjustment pattern' to a situation with very poor occupational opportunities (and a high degree of economic disorder) is using whatever chance is offered to get a job (using chance opportunities). This involves looking around for jobs, keeping good contacts with people who know something, and motivation as well as flexibility to accept whatever is offered. It can be understood very easily that this adjustment pattern was not relevant in the occupational situation for men around or past retirement age in an affluent society with (relatively) high pensions. On the other hand, in 1948 these men (about 45 years of age) did not react in an evasive manner to the occupational situation and they could not solve the problem by identifying with the aims and successes of their children or grandchildren.

Table I. Rank order of adjustment patterns to occupational problems as reported by men (born between 1900 and 1905) for 1948 and 1965

1948	1965
1 Achievement-oriented behavior	1 Achievement-oriented behavior
2 Adjustment to the institutional aspects of the situation	2 Identification with the aims and/or successes (sometimes failures) of children and grandchildren
3 Adjustment to the habits and/or needs of others	3 Seeking and/or cultivating social contacts
4 Establishing and/or cultivating social contacts	4 Accepting situation as it is
5 Using chance opportunities	5 Adjustment to the habits and/or needs of others
6 Active resistance against obstacles	6 Evasive reactions
7 Accepting situation as it is	7 Adjustment to the institutional aspects of the situation
8 Hope for help from others	8 Hope for help from others
9 To rely on others	9 Active resistance against others
10 Aggressive reaction	10 Depressive reaction
11 Asking others for help	11 Aggressive reaction
12 Depressive reaction	12 To rely on others
13 Resignation in favor of others	13 To disengage from situation
14 Identification with the aims and/or successes (sometimes failures) of children	14 Resignation in favor of others
15 Evasive reaction	15 Using chance opportunities

τ (Kendall II) = 0.276; $p > 5\%$.

The greatest contribution to the 'cognitive restructuration of the situation' in our aged subjects during the years of the study (1965–1973) was related to a group of reactions which we called 'identification with the achievements and aims of children'. Many of our low-income subjects told us, after they reported their economic situation: 'Well, I myself had poor luck, but my son (grandson, daughter, etc.) made it.' Their offspring's success was experienced as their own success. Even if the situation of the children or grandchildren was not extremely good, it could be perceived in a manner which provided satisfaction or helped in coping with feelings of dissatisfaction regarding the economic and/or occupational situation. Some of these reactions may be combined with cognitive distortions, but for many of our subjects the economic and occupational status of their offspring was not only a monetary asset but even more an aid in the cognitive restructuration of the own situation, especially regarding its economic aspects.

This process of restoring the emotional or cognitive balance, e.g. in light of discrepancies between desires and achieved goals, by identification with the status of offspring, is one example of a group of 'techniques', which can be defined as techniques of *'cognitive restructuration'*. This 'cognitive restructuration' of the situation is one of the main instruments for restoring the internal balance in aged persons who very often are faced with situations which can be changed in the way they are perceived, but not in reality. Besides 'identification with offspring's status' we could observe three other forms in our subjects: (a) positive interpretation of events (e.g., 'I am quite fine, if you compare my lot with that of poor Mr. X'); (b) revision of own expectations (e.g., 'well, as long as you are young you believe you must get everything, but when you get older you learn to enjoy whatever you have'), and (c) acceptance of the situation as it is (e.g., 'well, it could have been worse' or 'who knows what this will be good for? '). It is quite evident that this type of problem solving differs entirely from *achievement-oriented behavior,* which always involves some change in the external world.

There are some similarities between 'cognitive restructuration' and *'adjustment to the needs and habits of others'* (e. g. paying 'compliments', not talking too loud at home because of conflict with some neighbors). However, adjustment always remains an active effort which maintains a given goal whereas 'cognitive resturcturation' more often is related to situations which require resignation or insight into the unchangeable character of the situation. On the other hand, 'cognitive restructuration' is not identical with *'passive reaction'* or 'mood of general resignation', 'depressive reaction', or evasive behavior. Whereas these reactions preserve the unbalanced situation, 'cognitive restructuration' has the aim of restoring balance. This group of 'techniques' or 'problem-solving devices' certainly differs from a fifth group which includes different forms of *'assertive behavior'* like 'resistance to socially required demands' or of 'appealing to the next higher authority' (e. g. regarding pension).

Preliminary data available so far for ten subjects of each of the age/sex groups concerning consistency and change of these five problem-solving strategies in economic and occupational situations point to decreasing scores for achievement-oriented behavior from 1948 to 1965 and to consistency in scores from the first to the last MP (1965–1972). Whereas these trends were similar in all groups, mean scores for men are always higher by 1–1.5 points. This finding has to be interpreted with reference to the decrease in economic problems from 1948 to 1965 and the consolidation of this situation during the following years.

Whereas mean scores for achievement-oriented behavior are at the middle of the rating scales, they drop to 3–3.8 in men and to 1–2 in women. This finding means that achievement-oriented behavior can still contribute very much to economic balance in old age, but far less than before. This kind of 'strategy', however, was consistently more discernable than all of the remaining 'strategies'. This identifies our sample as a group of aged men and women who react to their problems in a rather active way. This statement is supported by the variability of scores for 'adjustment' in its different forms. Mean scores center around 2.5 in the four age/sex groups in 1948 and around 1.0 between MP I and MP V.

The trends for 'cognitive restructuration of the situation' differ in the sex groups. In both groups of men there is an increase from 1948 to 1972 (from 0.9 to 1.6). This would confirm our expectation that cognitive restructuration of the situation will become a major strategy for problem solving in situations which cannot be changed (loss of savings). But we have to mention a sex difference. In women, scores are rather consistent from 1948 to 1965 (from 0.8 to 1.0 in the older and from 1.7 to 1.9 in the younger age group) and decreased from MP I to MP V. On the other hand, we observed an increase in 'assertive behavior' from 1965 to 1973 in both women groups (from 0.5 to 1.2). This rising trend for 'assertive behavior' can be observed even more in both men groups (from 1.1 to 2.5. in the younger, from 0.4 to 1.25 in the older group).

'Passive reactions' got consistently low scores in the older age groups and the younger women group (0.2–0.4) at all MPs. Men of the cohort 1900–1905, who scored as low in 1948 and 1965, gave reports on their situation from 1965 to 1973 scoring for 'passive reactions' from 1.0 to 1.8.

Generally, we might state that the number of 'strategies' reported was rather low in the years of observation. We might predict a decisive increase in times of economic depression. Generally, more active strategies prevail, with 'active opposition' scoring higher with increasing age and achievement-oriented behavior scoring lower.

Whereas there are some indications that 'cognitive restructuration', as a strategy of solving problems which cannot be solved by changes in social (or biological, etc.) reality, will become more relevant with increasing age, we could not confirm this for the women groups. This may be explained by reference to how they perceived the situation. Apparently it was more often perceived as something which can be changed, whereas men 'knew about the realities of life'. This opinion would be supported by the increase of scores for 'assertive behavior'.

Generally we may state that the role of cognitive restructuring of the situation in adjustment to aging could not be assessed sufficiently within our study. We might find it represented more often in samples of disabled aged for whom this strategy might serve as the only 'successful' one. Furthermore, this type of problem solving may occur more often in those 'normal aging' samples in which distortion of the balance between self and social system may be reported more frequently. In any case, our findings lead us to expect that the ways of restoring balance between the aged and the biological-social systems cannot be reduced to one dimension like 'autonomy-dependency' (*Williams and Wirths,* 1965). As there are different ways of maintaining and restoring this balance, we might identify more patterns of aging or life-styles in terms of this focal developmental task in old age.

According to *Oesterreich* (1975), we can even define the difference between 'normal' and 'pathological' aging in terms of this balance between cognitive and motivational systems by processes of restructuring concepts of self and others and changing attitudes and expectations. His paper demonstrates how research on 'normal' and 'pathological' aging can be integrated if gerontology increasingly becomes conceived as the science of patterns of aging instead of a generalized development.

Concluding Remarks

The findings of our study as summarized in this volume are in agreement with those of most of the research groups who used community aged persons as subjects. They question a general correlation between calendar age and psychological change as defined by variables like intelligence, psychomotor performance and personality and point to influences of health, SES (education, occupation, income), ecology, degree of social integration and perception of self and others, etc.

One of the major conclusions to be drawn from this study is related to the definition of gerontology as a science of different forms or 'patterns' of aging and their biological, social, and ecological correlates.

Those who feel that differential approaches should replace or supplement generalizing tendencies in behavioral science may have expected a list of well-defined patterns as a result of our endeavors like those reported previously in this chapter. One of the main reasons why we do not summarize our findings by such a list is related to recent developments in personality theory. Any definition of a 'type' of aging is more or less closely related to a trait concept of personality. On the other hand, trait theories of personality have been questioned by interactionistic (*Rotter*), situationism (*Mischel,* 1969) and other (*Thomae,* 1968) approaches.

From these more recent trends in personality theory we should regard the different principles for classification of patterns of aging as instruments for the assessment of the individual life course in late adulthood. From our findings regarding consistency and change of psychological functioning and adjustment in old age we should define patterns of aging in terms of biological, social and perceptual-motivational processes. Patterns of this kind might support theoretical as well as applied research. Any kind of prediction of adjustment to aging and of planning services and support for the aged would require a systematic assessment of the different 'subsystems' which define the aging process in a given individual-environment interaction. There can be defined approximately ten of these subsystems.

(1) Nature-nurture constellation at the 'beginning' of the aging process (e. g. heredity, educational history, habits regarding physical and mental activity, nutrition, smoking, cultivating interests and social contacts).

(2) Recent changes in the biological system (health, sensory functions, primary process of aging, short-term memory, etc.).

(3) Recent changes in the social role system (retirement, loss of spouse, other relatives, friends, new friendships, 'substitute roles').

(4) Socioeconomic and ecological situation (e. g. income, social security, housing, transportation, availability of medical care, of preventive measures, etc.).

(5) Consistency and change in different aspects of cognitive functioning.

(6) Consistency and change in personality (activity, interest, mood, creativity, adjustment, ego control).

(7) Individual life space (self-concept, concept of 'significant others', perceived socioeconomic, political and historical situation, general belief-value systems (religion, attitude toward death).

(8) Life satisfaction or degree of attained balance between individual needs and perceived life situation.

(9) Capacity for restoring balance by 'active coping' (achievement-oriented behavior, adjustment, cognitive restructuring).

(10) 'Social competence' as a global measure for the individual's capacity to meet social and biological demands and the society's capacity to meet individual needs and capacities.

Patterns of aging (as defined from these ten 'dimensions' or 'subsystems' of the system 'aging individual') are outcomes of the complex interaction between these subsystems. In terms of this complex network there does not exist one way to 'successful' aging. Any recommendation for 'interventions' and services in support of successful aging has to be evaluated in terms of the great variability in which the balance of 'internal' and 'external' milieu can be disturbed and restored and in terms of the effects of this restoration for increased social competence of the aging individual.

References[1]

Adams, D. L.: Correlates of satisfaction among the elderly. Gerontologist *13:* 58–61 (1973).

Anastasi, A.: Länge des Schulbesuchs und Intelligenz; in *Weinert* Pädagogische Psychologie, pp. 524–528 (Kiepenheuer & Witsch, Köln 1967).

Anderson, B., jr. and Palmore, E.: Longitudinal evaluation of ocular function; in *Palmore* Normal aging. II, pp. 24–32 (Duke University Press, Durham 1974).

Angleitner, A.: Rigidität im Alter; phil. Diss. Bonn (1972).

Angleitner, A.: Faktorenanalytische Untersuchungen zum Konzept der Rigidität. Arch. Psychol. *125:* 73–104 (1973).

**Angleitner, A.:* Konstanz und Veränderlichkeit von Rigidität im Alter. actuelle gerontologie *4:* 1–8 (1974a).

**Angleitner, A.:* Changes in personality of older people over a 5-year period of observation. Gerontologia *20:* 179–185 (1974b).

Angleitner, A.; Rudinger, G.; Bierhoff, H. W. und Schmitz-Scherzer, R.: Einige Intelligenzmaße in ihrer Abhängigkeit von Schulbildung, Geschlecht, Alter und Gesundheit. actuelle gerontologie *3:* 163–179 (1973).

Angleitner, A.; Schmitz-Scherzer, R. und Rudinger, G.: Die Altersabhängigkeit der Persönlichkeit im Sinne von R. B. Cattell. actuelle gerontologie *1:* 721–729 (1971).

*Arbeitsgruppe Alternsforschung Bonn: Altern – psychologisch gesehen (Westermann, Braunschweig 1971).

Armor, D. J. and Couch, A. S.: Data-text primer. An introduction to computerized social data analysis (Free Press, New York 1972).

Ash, P.: Pre-retirement counseling. Gerontologist *6:* 61–64 (1966).

Atchley, R. C.: The social forces in later life. An introduction to social gerontology (Wadsworth, Belmont 1972).

Baer, D. M.: An age-irrelevant concept of development. Merrill-Palmer *16:* 230–245 (1970).

Baer, D. M.: The control of developmental process: why wait; in *Nesselroade and Reese* Life-span developmental psychology: methodological issues, pp. 187–196 (Academic Press, New York 1973).

Baeumler, G.: Zum altersbedingten psychischen Leistungsabbau mit Berücksichtigung der Stroop-Interferenzneigung. Psychol. Beitr. *11:* 34–67 (1969).

1 Titles with asterisk refer to publications from the Bonn Longitudinal Study of Aging.

Baldwin, A. L.: A cognitive theory of socialization; in *Goslin* Handbook of socialization theory and research, pp. 325–345 (Rand McNally, Chicago 1969).

Balinsky, B.: An analysis of mental factors of various age groups from nine to sixty. Genet. Psychol. Monogr. *23:* 192–234 (1941).

Baltes, P.: Longitudinal and cross-sectional sequences in the study of age and generation effects. Hum. Dev. *11:* 145–171 (1968).

Baltes, P. B.: Strategies for psychological intervention in old age. Gerontologist *13:* 4–38 (1973).

Baltes, P. B. and Goulet, L. R.: Life-span developmental psychology: status and issues; in *Goulet and Baltes* Life-span developmental psychology, theory and research, pp. 4–19 (Academic Press, New York 1970).

Baltes, P. B. and Goulet, L. R.: Explorations of developmental variables by manipulation and simulation of age differences in behavior. Hum. Dev. *14:* 149–170 (1971).

Baltes, P. B. and Labouvie, G. V.: Adult development of intellectual performance; description, explanation, and modification; in *Eisdorfer and Lawton* The psychology of adult development and aging (American Psychological Association, Washington 1973).

Baltes, P. B. and Nesselroade, J. R.: Multivariate longitudinal and cross-sectional sequences for analysing ontogenetic and generational change. Dev. Psychol. *2:* 163–168 (1970).

Baltes, P. B. and Nesselroade, J. R.: The developmental analysis of individual differences on multiple measures; in *Nesselroade and Reese* Life-span developmental psychology: methodological issues, pp. 219–252 (Academic Press, New York 1973).

Baltes, P. B.; Nesselroade, J. R.; Schaie, K. W., and Labouvie, E. W.: On a dilemma of regression effects in examining ability level-related differentials in ontogenetic patterns of intelligence. Dev. Psychol. *6:* 78–84 (1972).

Baltes, P. B. and Schaie, K. W.: Life-span developmental psychology: personality and socialization (Academic Press, New York 1973a).

Baltes, P. B. and Schaie, K. W.: On life-span developmental research paradigms; in *Baltes and Schaie* Live-span developmental psychology: personality and socialization; 366–396 (Academic Press, New York 1973b).

Baltes, P. B.; Schaie, K. W., and Nardi, A. H.: Age and experimental mortality in a seven-year longitudinal study of cognitive behavior. Dev. Psychol. *5:* 18–26 (1971).

Barker, R. G. and Barker, L.: Behavior units for the comparative study of culture; in *Kaplan* Studying personality across culture (Row Peterson, Evanston 1961).

Barker, R. G. and Barker, L. S.: Sixty-five and over; in *Williams, Tibbitts and Donahue* Processes of aging, pp. 246–272 (Atherton, New York 1963).

Baumrind, D.: Effects of authoritative control on child behavior. Child Dev. *37:* 886–907 (1974).

Becker, K.: Freizeit und Alter – Skizzierung einiger Aspekte. Z. Geront. *7:* 235–244 (1974).

Bedler, H. S.: Personal change in adult life; in *Neugarten* Middle age and aging, pp. 148–159 (University of Chicago Press, Chicago 1968).

Bell, B.; Rose, C. L. and Damon, A.: The veterans administration longitudinal study of healthy aging. Gerontologist *6:* 179–183 (1966).

Bellers, S. and Palmore, E.: Longevity in Turkey. Gerontologist *14:* 373–376 (1974).

Belson, W.: Volunteer bias in test-room groups. Publ. Opin. Q. *24:* 115–126 (1960).

Benny, M.; Gray, A. P., and Pear, R. H.: How people vote (Grove, New York 1956).

Bentler, P. M.: Assessment of developmental factor change at the individual and group level; in *Nesselroade and Reese* Life-span developmental psychology – methodological issues, pp. 145–166 (Academic Press, New York 1973).

Bereiter, C.: Some persisting dilemmas in the measurement of change; in *Harris* Problems in measuring change (University of Wisconsin Press, Madison 1963).

Berelson, B. R.; Lazarsfeld, P. F., and McPhee, W. N.: Voting (University of Chicago Press, Chicago 1954).

Berkowitz, B. and Green, R. E.: Changes in intellect with age. V. differential changes as functions of time interval and original score. J. genet. Psychol. *107:* 179–192 (1965).

Bijou, S. W.: Environment and intelligence: a behavioral analysis; in *Cancro* Contributions to intelligence (Grune & Stratton, New York 1971).

Birren, J. E.: Psychological aspects of aging. A. Rev. Psychol. *11:* 161–198 (1960).

Birren, J. E.: The psychology of aging (Prentice Hall, Englewood Cliffs 1964).

Birren, J. E.: Age changes in speed of behavior: its central nature and physiological correlates; in *Welford and Birren* Behavior, aging and the nervous system (Thomas, Springfield 1965).

Birren, J. E. and Botwinick, J. J.: Age differences in finger, jaw and foot reactions to auditory stimuli. J. Geront. *10:* 430–432 (1955).

Birren, J.; Botwinick, J.; Weiss, A., and Morrison, F. F.: Interrelations of mental and perceptual tests given to healthy elderly men; in *Birren, Butler et al.* Human aging, pp. 143–156 (National Institute of Mental Health, Bethesda 1963).

Birren, J. E.; Butler, R. N.; Greenhouse, S. W.; Sokoloff, L., and Yarrow, M. R.: Human aging: a biological and behavioral study (National Institute of Mental health, Bethesda 1963).

Birren, J. and Morrison, D. F.: Analysis of the WAIS subtests in relation to age and education. J. Geront. *16:* 363–369 (1961).

Birren, J. E. and Woodruff, D. S.: Human development over life-span through education; in *Baltes and Schaie* Life-span developmental psychology: personality and socialization, pp. 306–339 (Academic Press, New York 1973).

Birren, J.; Woodruff, D. R., and Bergman, S.: Research, demonstration, and training: issues and methodology in social gerontology. Gerontologist *12:* 49–83 (1972).

Bloom, B. S.: Stability and change in human characteristics (Wiley, New York 1964).

Blume, O.: Alte Menschen in der Großstadt (Schwartz, Göttingen 1962).

Bogue, D.: The population of the United States (Free Press, Glencoe 1959).

Bottenberg, E. H.: Kognitive Attitüden und Intelligenz. Psychol. Beitr. *12:* 415–446 (1970).

Botwinick, J.: Cognitive processes in maturity and old age (Springer, New York 1967).

Botwinick, J.: Geropsychology. A. Rev. Psychol. *21:* 239–272 (1970).

Botwinick, J. J.; Robbin, J. S., and Brinley, J. F.: Reorganization of perceptions with age. J. Geront. *14:* 85–88 (1959).

Bredenkamp, J.: Über Maße der praktischen Signifikanz. Z. Psychol. *177:* 310–318 (1970).

Brengelmann, J. C. und Brengelmann, L.: Deutsche Validierung von Fragebögen der Extraversion, neurotischen Tendenz und Rigidität. Z. exp. angew. Psychol. *7:* 291–331 (1960a).

Brengelmann, J. C. und Brengelmann, L.: Deutsche Validierung von Fragebögen dogmatischer und intoleranter Haltungen. Z. exp. angew. Psychol. *7:* 451–471 (1960b).

Britton, P. G.; Bergmann, K.; Kay, D. W., and Savage, R.: Mental state, cognitive functioning, physical health, and social class in the community aged. J. Geront. *22:* 517–521 (1967).

Britton, J. H. and Britton, J. O.: Survival of older adults and their personality and adjustment. Proc. 8th Int. Congr. Gerontology, vol. 2, p. 62 Washington (1969).

Bronson, W. C.: Central orientations; a study of behavior organization from childhood to adolescence. Child Dev. *37:* 125–155 (1966).

Bronson, W. C.: Adult derivates of emotional expressiveness and reactivity-control: developmental continuities from childhood to adulthood. Child Dev. *38:* 801–817 (1967).

Brown, R.: Social psychology (Free Press, New York 1965).

Bruhn, J. G.: An ecological perspective of aging. Gerontologist *11:* 318–321 (1971).

Buehler, C.: Der menschliche Lebenslauf als psychologisches Problem (1933); 2nd ed. (Verlag für Psychologie, Göttingen 1959).

Burgess, E. W.; Cavan, R. S., and Havighurst, R. J.: Your activities and attitudes; in *Havighurst and Albrecht* Older people, pp. 382–407 (Green and Company, New York 1953).

Buss, A. R.: An extension of developmental models that separate ontogenetic changes and cohort differences. Psychol. Bull. *80:* 466–479 (1973).

Buss, A. R.: A recursive-nonrecursive factor model and developmental causal networks. Hum. Dev. *17:* 139–151 (1974a).

Buss, A. R.: A general developmental model for interindividual differences, intraindividual differences, and intraindividual changes. Devl Psychol. *10:* 70–78 (1974b).

Buss, A. R.: Multivariate model of quantitative, structural, and quantistructural ontogenetic change. Devl Psychol. *10:* 190–203 (1974c).

Buss, A. R.: More on the age x cohort developmental models: Reply to Labouvie. Psychol. Bull. *82:* 165–169 (1975).

Busse, E. W.: Theories of aging; in *Busse and Pfeiffer* Behavior and adaptation in late life, pp. 11–32 (Little, Brown, Boston 1969).

Busse, E. W.; Dovenmuehle, R. M., and Brown, R. G.: Psychoneurotic reactions of the aged; in *Palmore,* Normal Aging pp. 75–83 Duke University Press, Durham (1970).

Campbell, D. T. and Stanley, J. C.: Experimental and quasi-experimental designs for research on teaching; in *Gage* Handbook of research on teaching, chap. 5 (Rand McNally, Chicago 1963).

Cattell, R. B.: The theory of fluid and crystallized intelligence: a critical experiment. J. educ. Psychol. *54:* 1–22 (1963).

Cattell, R. B.: Scientific analysis of personality (Penguin Books, London 1965).

Cattell, R. B.: Separating endogenous, exogenous, ecogenic and epogenic component curves in developmental data. Devl Psychol. *2:* 163–172 (1970).

Charles, D.: Historical antecedents of life-span developmental psychology; in *Goulet and Baltes* Life-span developmental psychology, pp. 24–51 (Academic Press, New York 1970).

Chebotarev, D. F.: Longevity and aging processes. Proc. 8th Int. Congr. Gerontology, vol. 5, p. 382 (Washington 1969).

Chown, S. M.: Age and the rigidities. J. Geront. *16:* 353–362 (1961).

Chown, S. M.: Human ageing (Penguin Books, London 1972).

Chown, S. M. and Heron, A.: Psychological aspects of aging in man. A. Rev. Psychol. *16:* 417–450 (1965).

Clark, A. M.: Genetic factors associated with aging; in *Strehler* Advances in gerontological research, pp. 207–255 (Academic Press, New York 1964).

Coerper, C.; Hagen, W. und Thomae, H.: Deutsche Nachkriegskinder (Thieme, Stuttgart 1954).

Coleman, J. S.: The mathematical study of change; in *Blalock, jr. and Blalock* Methodology in social research, pp. 428–478 (McGraw-Hill, New York 1968).

Correll, R. E. and Rokosz, J. E.: Some correlates of WAIS performance in the elderly. J. Geront. *21:* 544–549 (1966).

Cronbach, L. J. and Furby, L.: How should we measure change – or should we? Psychol. Bull. *74:* 68–80 (1970).

Cronbach, L. J.; Gleser, G. C.; Nanda, H., and Rajaratnam, N.: The dependability of behavioral measurements (Wiley, New York 1972).

Cumming, E. and Henry, W. E.: Growing old: the process of disengagement (Basic Books, New York 1961).

Cunningham, W. R.; Clayton, U. Z., and Overton, W.: Fluid and crystallized intelligence in adulthood and old age. J. Geront. *30:* 53–55 (1975).

Eisdorfer, C.: The WAIS performance of the aged: a retest evaluation. J. Geront. *18:* 169–172 (1963).

Eisdorfer, C.: Arousal and performance: experiments in verbal learning and a tentative theory; in *Talland* Human aging and behavior, pp. 189–214 (Academic Press, New York 1968).

Elashoff, J. D.: Analysis of covariance: a delicate instrument. Am. Educ. Res. J. *6:* 383–401 (1969).

Emmerich, W.: Personality development and concepts of structure. Child Dev. *39:* 671–690 (1968).

**Erlemeier, N.:* Rorschachbefunde im höheren Alter. Z. Geront. *1:* 296–310 (1968).

**Erlemeier, N. und Angleitner, A.:* Untersuchungen zur 'Rigidität' im höheren Alter. Z. Geront. *4:* 194–207 (1971).

Feifel, H.: Judgment of time in younger and older persons. J. Geront. *12:* 71–74 (1957).

Felstein, I.: Living to be a hundred (David & Charles, Newton Abbot 1973).

Fink, H. H.: The relationship of time perspective to age, institutionalization and activity. J. Geront. *12:* 414–417 (1957).

Fischer, G. und Roppert, J.: Bemerkungen zu einem Verfahren der Transformationsanalyse. Arch. Psychol. *116:* 92–97 (1964).

Fisher, J.: Competence, effectiveness, intellectual functioning, and aging. Gerontologist *13:* 62–68 (1973).

Foulds, G. A. and Raven, C. J.: Normal changes in mental abilities of adults as age advances. J. ment. Sci. *94:* 133–142 (1948).

Franke, H.: Das Wesen der Polypathie bei 100jährigen. Ber. Symp. dt. Ges. Gerontologie über diagnostische und therapeutische Probleme der Multimorbidität in der Geriatrie (Nürnberg 1971a).

Franke, H.: Kriterien der überdurchschnittlichen Lebenserwartung. Medsche Klin. *66:* 896 (1971b).

Franke, H.: Das Wesen der Polypathie bei 100jährigen. Ber. Symp. dt. Ges. Gerontologie, Nürnberg; in *Schubert und Strömer* Schwerpunkte in der Geriatrie (Banaschewski, München 1973).

Franke, H.; Bracharz, H. und Gall, L.: Frühere Lebensweisen von 100jährigen und Älteren. Ber. Symp. dt. Ges. Gerontologie, Nürnberg (Banaschewski, München 1973).

Franke, H.; Bracharz, H.; Laas, H. und Moll, E.: Studien an 148 Hundertjährigen. Dt. med. Wschr. *95:* 1590 (1970).

Franke, H. und Schmitt, I.: Hundertjährige (Verlag der Fränkischen Gesellschaftsdruckerei, Würzburg 1971).

Fröhlich, W. D.; Becker, J. P.; Bengtson, V. L., and Bigot, A.: The problem of cross-national reliability in ratings, some tentative approaches and findings; in *Havighurst et al.* Adjustment to retirement. A cross-national study, pp. 18–34 (Van Gorcum, Assen 1969).

Furby, L.: Interpreting regression toward the mean in developmental research. Dev. Psychol. *8:* 172 (1973).

Gleser, G. C.; Cronbach, L. J., and Rajaratnam, N.: Generalizability scores influenced by multiple sources of variance. Psychometrika *30:* 395–418 (1965).

Goldfarb, A.: Predicting mortality in the institutionalized aged. Archs gen. Psychiat. *21:* 172–176 (1969).

Gottesman, L.E.: Milieu treatment of the aged in institutions. Gerontologist *13/1:* 23–27 (1973).

Granick, S.: Cognitive aspects of longevity; in *Palmore and Jeffers* Prediction of life span (Lexington Books, Lexington 1971).

Granick, S. and Birren, J. E.: Cognitive functioning of survivors versus non-survivors: 12 years follow-up of healthy aged. Proc. 8th Int. Congr. Gerontology, vol. 2, p. 67 (Washington 1969).

Granick, S. and Friedman, A. S.: The effect of education in the decline of test performance with age. J. Geront. *22:* 191–195 (1967).

Granick, S. and Friedman, A. S.: Educational experience and the maintenance of intellectual functioning by the aged: an overview; in *Jarvik, Eisdorfer and Blum* Intellectual functioning in adults: psychological and biological influences (Springer, New York 1973).

Granick, S. and Patterson, R. D.: Human aging. II. An eleven year follow-up biomedical and behavioral study. DHEW Publication, No. (HSM) 71–9037 (US Government Printing Office, Washington 1971).

Green, R. F.: Age-intelligence relationships between ages sixteen and sixty-four: a rising trend. Dev. Psychol. *1:* 618–627 (1969).

Groffmann, K. J.: Life-span developmental psychology in Europe: past and present; in *Goulet and Baltes* Life-span developmental psychology, pp. 54–67 (Academic Press, New York 1970).

**Grombach, H. H.:* Possibilities and problems of longitudinal analysis by comparisons of factor-structure and factor-scores applied to a set of behavioral data. Paper read at 2nd Biennial Meeting of the ISSBD (Ann Arbor 1973).

**Grombach, H. H.:* Konstanz und Variabilität von Persönlichkeitsmerkmalen; phil. Diss. Bonn (1975).

Hagen, W. und Thomae, H.: Deutsche Nachkriegskinder (Barth, München 1962).

Haranghy, L. E.; Bereyi, E., and Laslo, B.: Gerontological studies on Hungarian centenarians (Akademiai Kiado Alkotmany, Budapest 1965).

Harwood, E. and Naylor, G. F. K.: Changes in the constitution of the WAIS intelligence pattern with advancing age. Aust. J. Psychol. *23:* 297–303 (1971).

Haug, G.: Vom Tätigsein im Alter – Forderungen an Wirtschaft und Sozialarbeit. Z. Geront. *7:* 245–254 (1974).

Havighurst, R. J.: Research on the developmental-task concept. Sch. Rev. *63:* 215–223 (1956).

Havighurst, R. J.: Successful aging; in *Tibbitts and Donahue* Processes of aging, pp. 299–320 (Williams, New York 1963).

Havighurst, R. J.: Disengagement personality and life satisfaction in the later years; in *Hansen* Age with a future, pp. 419–425 (Munksgaard, Kopenhagen 1964).

Havighurst, R. J.: Developmental tasks and education; 3rd ed. (McKay, New York 1972).

Havighurst, R. J.: History of developmental psychology: socialization and personality development through the life-span; in *Baltes and Schaie* Life-span developmental psychology – personality and socialization, pp. 4–23 (Academic Press, New York 1973).

Havighurst, R. J.: Life style transitions related to personality after age fifty (unpublished, 1975).

Havighurst, R. J. and DeVries, A.: Life styles and free time activities of retirement. Hum. Dev. *12:* 34–54 (1969).

Havighurst, R. J.; Munnichs, J. M.; Neugarten, B. and Thomae, H.: Adjustment to retirement. A cross-national study (Van Gorcum, Assen 1969).

Havighurst, R. J.; Neugarten, B., and Tobin, S.: Disengagement and patterns of aging. Gerontologist *4:* 24 (1964).

Havighurst, R. J.; Neugarten, B., and Tobin, S. H.: Disengagement and patterns of aging; in

Neugarten Middle age and aging, pp. 161–172 (University of Chicago Press, Chicago 1968).

Hays, W.L.: Statistics for the social sciences; 2nd ed. (Holt, Rinehart & Winston, London 1973).

Heegner, F.: Zum Problem des Reaktionsvermögens. Zentbl. Verk.-Med. *3:* 1–14 (1957).

Heise, D. R.: Separating reliability and stability in test-retest correlation; in *Blalock, jr.* Causal models in the social sciences (Macmillan, London 1971).

Helson, H.: Adaptation level theory (Wiley, New York 1964).

Henry, W. E.: The theory of intrinsic disengagement; in *Hansen* Age with a future, pp. 415–418 (Munksgaard, Copenhagen 1964).

Heron, A. and Chown, S. M.: Psychological aspects of ageing in man. A. Rev. Psychol. *7:* 349–364 (1956).

Herrmann, T.: Lehrbuch der empirischen Persönlichkeitsforschung (Verlag für Psychologie, Göttingen 1969).

Herrmann, T.: Persönlichkeitsmerkmale – Bestimmung und Verwendung in der psychologischen Wissenschaft (Kohlhammer, Stuttgart 1973).

Holland, H. C.: The spiral after-effect and the rigidity – dysthymia hypothesis. Acta psychol. *22:* 100–108 (1964).

Holtmeier, H. J.: Die Ernährung des alternden Menschen (Thieme, Stuttgart 1968).

Honzik, M. P.: Environmental correlates of mental growth: prediction from the family setting at 21 months. Child Dev. *38:* 337–364 (1967).

Horn, J. L.: Organization of data on life-span development of human abilities; in *Goulet and Baltes* Life-span developmental psychology: research and theory, pp. 424–464 (Academic Press, New York 1970).

Horn, J. L. and Cattell, R. B.: Age differences in primary mental ability factors. J. Geront. *21:* 210–220 (1966).

Horn, J. L. and Cattell, R. B.: Age differences in fluid and crystallized intelligence. Acta psychol. *26:* 107–129 (1967).

Hoyos, C.: Die psychophysische Belastbarkeit als diagnostische Kategorie der Kraftfahrtauglichkeit. Z. exp. angew. Psychol. *7:* 226–243 (1960a).

Hoyos, C.: Diskussionsbemerkung zu "Psychometrischer Ausbau der Kieler Belastungsprobe für die klinisch-psychologische Diagnostik", Psychol. Praxis, vol. 4, pp. 122–124 (Karger, Basel 1960b).

Hulicka, I. M.: Age changes and age differences in memory functioning. Gerontologist *7:* 46–69 (1967).

Humphrey, L. G.: Theory of intelligence; in *Cancro* Contributions to intelligence (Grune & Stratton, New York 1971).

Jarvik, L.F.: Biological differences in intellectual functioning. Vita hum. *5:* 195–203 (1962).

Jarvik, L. F.: Survival and psychological aspects of aging in man; in *Woolhouse* Aspects of the biology of aginy. Symp. Soc. Exp. Biology (Cambridge University Press, Cambridge 1967).

Jarvik, L. F. and Blum, J. E.: Cognitive decline as predictors of mortality in twin pairs; in *Palmore and Jeffers* Prediction of life span, pp. 199–212 (Lexington Books, 1971).

Jarvik, L. F.; Eisdorfer, C., and Blum, J. E.: Intellectual functioning in adults (Springer, New York 1973).

Jarvik, L. F. and Falek, A.: Intellectual stability and survival in the aged. J. Geront. *18:* 173–176 (1963).

Jeffers, F. C. and Nicols, C. R.: The relationship of activities and attitudes to physical well-being in older people; in *Palmore* Normal aging. I, pp. 304–309 (Duke University Press, Durham 1970).

Jones, H. E.: Consistency and change in early maturity. Vita hum. *1:* 43–51 (1958).

Jones, H. E.: Intelligence and problem solving; in *Birren* Handbook of aging, pp. 700–738 (Rand McNally, Chicago 1959).

Kagan, J.: American longitudinal research on psychological development. Child Dev. *35:* 1–32 (1964).

Kastenbaum, R.: New thoughts on old age (Springer, New York 1964).

Kastenbaum, R. and Durkee, N.: Elderly people view old age; in *Kastenbaum* New thoughts on old age, pp. 250–262 (Springer, New York 1964).

Katz, H.: Vergleichsuntersuchung zur Reaktionszeit und tachistoskopischen Auffassungsleistung bei weiblichen und männlichen Studierenden; unveröffentlichte psychologische Vorexamensarbeit Bonn (1969).

Klausner, S. Z.: On man in his environment (Jossey-Bass, San Francisco 1971).

Klausner, S. Z.: Life-span environmental psychology: methodological issues; in *Baltes and Schaie* Life-span developmental psychology: personality and socialization, pp. 72–97 (Academic Press, New York 1973).

Kleemeier, R. W.: Aging and leisure (Wiley, New York 1961).

Klonoff, H. and Kennedy, M.: A comparative study of cognitive functioning in old age. J. Geront. *21:* 239–243 (1966).

Kottenhoff, H.: Psychometrischer Ausbau der Kieler Belastungsprobe für die klinisch-psychologische Diagnostik. Psychol. Praxis, vol. 3, pp. 303–313 (Karger, Basel 1959).

Kuehn, D. und Plagemann, K.: Probleme der Altersfreizeit in der kommunalen Sozialplanung. Z. Geront *7:* 288–303 (1974).

Kuhlen, R. G.: Age and intelligence. Vita hum. *6:* 56–64 (1963).

Kuhlen, R. G.: Personality change with age; in *Worchel and Byrne* Personality change, pp. 524–556 (Springer, New York 1964).

Kuypers, I. A. and Bengston, K. L.: Social breakdown and comptetence. A normal model of aging. Hum. Dev. *16:* 181–201 (1973).

Labouvie, E. W.: An extension of developmental models: a reply to Buss. Psychol. Bull. *82:* 165–169 (1975).

Lambrev, J.: Untersuchung der Langlebigkeit in Bulgarien. Godisnik na medicinskijy facultet. Plovdivski Univ. Paisi Chilendazski Plovdiv, vol. 5, p. 102 (1951).

**Langermann-Erlenkamp, U.v.:* Reaktionsformen auf Belastungssituationen bei älteren Menschen; phil. Diss. Bonn (1970).

Lawton, M. P.: Ecology and aging; in *Pastalan and Carson* Spatial behavior of older people, pp. 40–67 (Institute of Gerontology, Ann Arbor 1970).

Lawton, M. P. and Nahemow, L.: Ecology and the aging process; in *Eisdorfer and Lawton* The psychology of adult development and aging, pp. 619–674 (American Psychological Association, Washington 1973).

Lawton, A. H. and Rich, T. A.: Ecology and gerontology: an introduction. Gerontologist *8:* 76–77 (1968).

Lazarus, R. S.: Personality and adjustment (Prentice Hall, Englewood Cliffs 1963).

Lazarus, R. S.: Psychological stress and the coping process (McGraw-Hill, New York 1966).

Leeper, R.: Some needed developments in the motivational theory of emotions; in *Levine* Nebraska Symp. on Motivation, pp. 25–122, (University of Nebraska Press, Lincoln 1965).

**Lehr, U.:* Attitudes toward the future. Hum. Dev. *10:* 230–238 (1967).

Lehr, U.: Frau im Beruf. Eine psychologische Analyse der weiblichen Berufsrolle (Athenäum, Frankfurt 1969).

Lehr, U.: Institutionalisierung älterer Menschen als psychologisches Problem – Ergebnisse der empirischen Forschung. Ber. Dt. Ges. Gerontologie, pp. 344–352 (Steinkopff, Darmstadt 1970).

Lehr, U.: Zur Psychologie des Alterns – Stereotypien und Erkenntnisse. actuelle gerontologie *1:* 17–24 (1971a).

Lehr, U.: Psycho-gerontologische Forschung in Deutschland – Rückblick und Ausblick. Z. Geront. *4:* 1–7 (1971b).

Lehr, U.: Psychologie des Alterns (UTB, Heidelberg 1972).

Lehr, U.: Gerontologie – ein Modell interdisziplinärer Forschung und Lehre? actuelle gerontologie *3:* 391–397 (1973).

Lehr, U.: Alter und Rehabilitation – psychologische Aspekte; in *Böhlau* Alter und Rehabilitation, pp. 87–99 (Schattauer, Stuttgart 1974).

Lehr, U. and Dreher, G.: Determinants of attitudes toward retirement; in *Havighurst, Munnichs, Neugarten and Thomae* Adjustment to retirement. A cross-national study, pp. 116–137 (Van Gorcum, Assen 1969).

**Lehr, U. und Merker, H.:* Jugend von heute in der Sicht des Alters. Ber. 4. Kongr. Dt. Ges. Gerontologie, pp. 255–267 (Steinkopff, Darmstadt 1970).

**Lehr, U. and Rudinger, G.:* Consistency and change of social participation in old age. Hum. Dev. *12:* 255–267 (1969).

**Lehr, U. und Rudinger, G.:* Strukturen der sozialen Teilhabe im höheren Lebensalter. Z. Geront. *4:* 81–88 (1970).

**Lehr, U., Schmitz-Scherzer, R. und Thomae, H.:* Psychologischer Status, subjektiver Gesundheitszustand und internistischer Befund. Ärztl. Prax., Wien *90:* 4393–4401 (1972).

**Lehr, U. und Schmitz-Scherzer, R.:* Psychosoziale Korrelate der Langlebigkeit. Acta geront. *4:* 261–268 (1974).

Lehr, U. und Thomae, H.: Eine Längsschnittuntersuchung bei 30–40jährigen Angestellten. Vita hum. *1:* 100–110 (1958).

Lehr, U. und Thomae, H.: Konflikt, seelische Belastung und Lebensalter (Westdeutscher Verlag, Opladen 1965).

Lewin, K.: Field theory and experiment in social psychology. Am. J. Sociol. *44:* 868–896 (1939).

Lewin, K.: Feldtheorie in den Sozialwissenschaften (Huber, Bern 1963).

Libow, L. S.: Interaction of medical, biologic, and behavioral factors on aging, adaptation, and survival: an 11 year longitudinal study. Geriatrics *29:* 75–88 (1974).

Lieberman, M. A.: Psychological correlates of impending death: some preliminary observations. J. Geront. *20:* 181–190 (1965).

Lieberman, M. A.; Prock, U. N., and Tobin, S.: Psychological effects of institutionalization. J. Geront. *23:* 343–353 (1968).

Lienert, G. A. and Krauth, J.: Configural frequency analysis as a statistical tool for defining types. Educ. psychol. Measur. *35:* 231–238 (1975).

Liese, L.: Vergleichsuntersuchung zur Relationsgeschwindigkeit fünfzehnjähriger Jungen und Mädchen; unveröffentlichte psychologische Vorexamensarbeit Bonn (1972).

Lindquist, E. F.: Design and analysis of experiments in psychology and education (Houghton Mifflin, Boston 1953).

Loeb, M. B.; Pincus, A., and Mueller, B. J.: A framework for viewing adjustment in aging. Gerontologist *6:* 178–185 (1966).

Loewe, H.: Einführung in die Lernpsychologie des Erwachsenenalters (VEB Volk und Wissen, Berlin 1970).

Looft, W. R.: Socialization and personality throughout the life-span: an examination of contemporary psychological approaches; in *Baltes and Schaie* Life-span developmental psychology: personality and socialization, pp. 26–52 (Academic Press, New York 1973).

Lord, F. M.: Elementary models for measuring change; in *Harris* Problems in measuring change, pp. 21–38 (University of Wisconsin Press, Madison 1963).

Lorge, I.: The influence of the tests upon the nature of mental decline as a function of age. J. educ. Psychol. *27:* 100–110 (1936).

Lowe, F. E. and McCormick, T. C.: Some survey sampling biases. Publ. Opin. Q. *19:* 303–315 (1955).

Luchins, A. S. and Luchins, E. A.: Rigidity of behavior. (University of Oregon, Oregon 1959).

Maas, H. S. and Kuypers, J. A.: From thirty to seventy. A forty year longitudinal study of adult life styles and personality (Jossey-Bass, San Francisco 1974).

Maddox, G.: Activity and morale: a longitudinal study of selected elderly subjects. Social forces *42:* 195–204 (1963).

Maddox, G. L.: Disengagement theory: a critical evaluation. Gerontologist *4:* 80–83 (1964).

Maddox, G. L.: Fact and artifact: evidence bearing on disengagement theory. Hum. Dev. *8:* 117–130 (1965).

Maddox, G. L.: Self-assessment of health status; in *Palmore* Normal aging, pp. 350–362 (Duke University Press, Durham 1970).

Maddox, G. L. and Eisdorfer, C.: Zusammenhänge zwischen Aktivität und Stimmung bei älteren Menschen. Social Forces *40:* 254–260 (1963); in *Thomae und Lehr* Altern – Probleme und Tatsachen (Reader), pp. 235–282 (Akademische Verlagsgesellschaft, Frankfurt 1968).

**Mathey, F. J.:* Reaktionen auf eine Belastungssituation im höheren Alter, vol. 1, pp. 223–227 (Deutsche Gesellschaft für Gerontologie, Darmstadt 1968).

**Mathey, F. J.:* Längsschnittuntersuchung zur Frage der psychophysischen Leistungsfähigkeit im höheren Alter, vol. 3, pp. 254–262, (Deutsche Gesellschaft für Gerontologie, Darmstadt 1970).

**Mathey, F. J.:* Psychische Reaktionen auf experimentelle Belastungssituationen – Ergebnisse longitudinaler Studien. actuelle gerontologie *1:* 103–109 (1971).

McFarlane, J. W.: Studies in child guidance. I. Methodology of data collection and organization. Monogr. Soc. Res. Child Dev. *3:* 1–254 (1938).

Medvedev, Z. A.: Aging and longevity – new approaches and new perspectives. Gerontologist *15:* 196–201 (1975).

Meresko, R.; Mandel, R.; Schontz, F. C. and Morrow, W. R.: Rigidity of attitudes regarding personal habits and its psychological correlates. J. abnorm. soc. Psychol. *49:* 89–93 (1954).

**Merker, H. M.:* Generations-Gegensätze. Eine empirische Erkundungsstudie über die Einstellung Erwachsener zur Jugend (Thesen-Verlag, Darmstadt 1973).

Mierke, K.: Wille und Leistung (Verlag für Psychologie, Göttingen 1955).

Mischel, W.: Continuity and change in personality. Am. Psychol. *24:* 1012–1018 (1969).

Moers, M.: Die Entwicklungsphasen des menschlichen Lebens (Henn, Ratingen 1953).

Mol, F. und Wimmers, M.: "Fluid" Intelligenz im Alter. actuelle gerontologie *1:* 159–165 (1971).

Monthofer, W.: Zur Belastbarkeit älterer Menschen – ein kasuistischer Längsschnittvergleich; unveröffentlichte psychologische Vorexamensarbeit Bonn (1970).

Moriwaki, S. Y.: The affect balance scale: a validity study with aged samples. J. Geront. *29:* 73–78 (1974).

Moss, M. A. and Kagan, J.: Report on personality consistency and change from the Fels longitudinal study. Vita hum. *7:* 127–138 (1964).

Mueller, H. F.; Grad, B. and Engelsmann, F.: Biological and psychological predictors of survival in psychogeriatric population. J. Geront. *30:* 47–52 (1975).

Munnichs, J. M. A.: Old age and finitude (Karger, Basel 1966).
Munnichs, J. M. A.: Die Frau um die Menopause. Z. Geront. *8:* 96–108 (1975).
Natsoulas, T.: Interpreting perceptual reports. Psychol. Bull. *70:* 575–591 (1968).
Nehrcke, F. M.: Age, sex, and educational differences in syllogistic reasoning. J. Geront. *27:* 466–470 (1972).
Nesselroade, J. R.: Application of multivariate strategies to problems of measuring and structuring long-term change; in *Goulet and Baltes* Life-span developmental psychology, pp. 194–207 (Academic Press, New York 1970).
Nesselroade, J. R.: Note on the 'longitudinal factor analysis' model. Psychometrika *37:* 187–191 (1972).
Nesselroade, J. R.: Faktorenanalyse von Kreuzprodukten zur Beschreibung von Veränderungsphänomenen (change). Z. exp. angew. Psychol. *20:* 92–106 (1973).
Nesselroade, J. R. and Baltes, P. B.: A study of ontogenetic and generational change in adolescent personality by means of multivariate longitudinal sequences: phase II. Final report project No. 1–0148 (US Department of Health, Education and Welfare, Washington 1973).
Nesselroade, J. R. and Cable, D.: 'Sometimes, it's okay to factor difference scores' – The separation of state and trait anxiety. Multivar. Behav. Res. *4:* 273–282 (1974).
Nesselroade, J. R. and Reese, H. W.: Life-span developmental psychology: methodological issues (Academic Press, New York 1973).
Nesselroade, J. R.; Schaie, K. W., and Baltes, P. B.: Ontogenetic and generational components of structural and quantitative change in adult cognitive behavior. J. Geront. *27:* 222–228 (1972).
Neugarten, B. L.: Middle age and aging (University of Chicago Press, Chicago 1968).
Neugarten, B. L.: Introduction to the symposium: models and methods for the study of life cycle. Hum. Dev. *14:* 81–86 (1971).
Neugarten, B. L.: Personality change in late life: a developmental perspective; in *Eisdorfer and Lawton* The psychology of adult development and aging, pp. 311–338 (American Psychological Association, Washington 1973).
Neugarten, B. L. and Havighurst, R. J.: Disengagement reconsidered in a cross-national context; in *Havighurst et al.* Adjustment to retirement, pp. 138–146 (Van Goreum, Assen 1969).
Neugarten, B. L.; Havighurst, R. J., and Tobin, S. Personality and patterns of aging. Tijdschr. psychol. Kting Nijmessgse Univ. *13:* 249–256 (1965).
Newell, D. S.: Social-structural evidence for disengagement; in *Cumming and Henry* Growing old: the process of disengagement, pp. 37–74 (Basic Books, New York 1961).
Oesterreich, K.: Zum Begriff der Norm in der Psychiatrie des Alterns. Nervenarzt *46:* 285–290 (1975).
**Olbrich, E.:* Veränderungen der Sozialkontakte und Anpassungsprobleme im Alter, actuelle gerontologie *4:* 767–770 (1974).
**Olbrich, E.:* Soziale Teilhabe im Alter; phil. Diss. Bonn (in Vorbereitung, 1975).
**Opgenoorth, W. P.:* Dimensionen des subjektiven Lebensraumes im höheren Alter; phil. Diss. Bonn (1971).
**Opgenoorth, W. und Thomae, H.:* Die Lebenssituation der älteren Menschen in subjektiver Sicht. Z. Geront. *3:* 210–215 (1970).
Orbens, H.: Erfahrungen beim Aufbau einer kommunalen Altenhilfe in einer süddeutschen Mittelstadt. Z. Geront. *7:* 304–311 (1974).
Overton, W. F. and H. W. Reese: Models of development: methodological implications; in *Nesselroade and Reese* Life-span developmental psychology: methodologicalisms, pp. 65–86 (Academic Press, New York 1973).

Owens, W. A.: Age and mental abilities, a longitudinal study. Genet. Psychol. Monogr. *48:* 3–54 (1953).

Owens, W. A.: Age and mental abilities: a second adult follow-up. J. educ. Psychol. *57:* 311–325 (1966).

Palmore, E.: The effects of aging on activities and attitudes. Gerontologist *8:* 259–263 (1968).

Palmore, E.: Physical, mental and social factors in predicting longevity. Gerontologist *9:* 103–108 (1969a).

Palmore, E.: Predicting longevity: a follow-up controlling for age. Gerontologist *9:* 247–253 (1969b).

Palmore, E.: Sociological aspects of aging; in *Busse and Pfeiffer* Behavior and adaptation in later life, pp. 33–69 (Little, Brown, Boston 1969c).

Palmore, E.: Normal aging (Duke University Press, Durham 1970).

Palmore, E.: Normal aging. II (Duke University Press, Durham 1974a).

Palmore, E.: Predicting longevity: a new method; in *Palmore* Normal aging. II (Duke University Press, Durham 1974b).

Palmore, E. and Jeffers, F.: Prediction of life span (Lexington Books, Lexington 1971).

Palmore, E. and Luikart, H.: Life satisfaction; in *Palmore* Normal aging. II, pp. 184–200 (Duke University Press, Durham 1974).

Parsons, T. and Shils, E. A. (Eds): Toward a general theory of action (University Press, Cambridge 1951).

Peters, G. R.: Self-conceptions of the aged, age identification, and aging. Gerontologist *11:* 69–73 (1971).

Pfeiffer, E.: Short-term vs. long-term survival in old age: physical, psychological and social correlates in two polar groups. Proc. 8th Int. Congr. on Gerontology, Washington, vol. 2, p. 48 (1969).

**Puschner, I.:* Daseinsthemen in verschiedenen Lebensaltern. Z. Geront. *1:* 311–327 (1968).

**Puschner, I.: Schreiner, M. und Tismer, K. G.:* Expansion und Restriktion in der Lebensthematik älterer Menschen. Ber. 1. Kongr. Dt. Ges. Gerontologie, pp. 204–214 (Steinkopff, Darmstadt 1968).

Radke-Yarrow, M.: Appraising environment; in *Williams, Tibbits and Donahue* Processes of aging, vol. 1, pp. 246–272 (Atherton, New York 1963).

Raven, J. C.: Guide to using the coloured progressive matrices; revised order 1956 (Lewis, London 1963).

Reichard, S.; Livson, F., and Petersen, P. G.: Aging and personality (Willy, New York 1962).

Reinert, G.: Comparative factor analytic studies of intelligence throughout the human lifespan; in *Goulet and Baltes* Life-span developmental psychology: research and theory (Academic Press, New York 1970).

Richardson, A.: Social and medical correlates of survival among octogenarians. J. Geront. *28:* 207–215 (1973).

Riegel, K. F.: Research designs in the study of aging and the prediction of retest – resistance and death. Proc. 8th Int. Congr. on Gerontology, pp. 455–457 (International Gerontological Society, Washington 1969).

Riegel, K. F. and Riegel, R. M.: A study on changes of attitudes and interests during later years of life. Vita hum. *3:* 177–206 (1960).

Riegel, K. F. and Riegel, R. M.: Development, drop and death. Dev. Psychol. *6:* 306–319 (1972).

Riegel, K. F.; Riegel, R. M., and Meyer, G.: Sociopsychological factors of aging: a cohort-sequential analysis. Hum. Dev. *10:* 27–56 (1967).

Riegel, K. F.; Riegel, R. M. und Skiba, G.: Untersuchung der Lebensbedingungen, Gewohnheiten und Anpassung älterer Menschen in Norddeutschland. Vita hum. *5:* 204–247 (1962).

Riegel, R. M.: Faktorenanalysen des "Hamburg-Wechsler-Intelligenztests für Erwachsene" (HAWIE) für die Altersstufen 20–34, 35–49, 50–64 und 65 Jahre und älter. Diagnostica *6:* 41–66 (1960).

Riegel, R. M. und Riegel, K. F.: Standardisierung des Hamburg-Wechsler-Intelligenztests (HAWIE) für die Altersstufen über 50 Jahre. Diagnostica *5:* 97–129 (1959).

Ries, W.: Der Flimmerfrequenz-Test in Abhängigkeit von Alter und Geschlecht. Z. Altersforsch. *14:* 318–326 (1960).

**Roeder, S.:* Ein Vergleich von HAWIE- und RAVEN-Leistungen bei älteren Menschen; unveröffentlichte Vorexamensarbeit Bonn (1971).

Rogers, C. R.: Die klient-bezogene Gesprächstherapie (Kindler, München 1973).

Rokeach, M.; McGovney, W. C., and Denny, M. R.: A distinction between dogmatic and rigid thinking. J. abnorm. soc. Psychol. *51:* 87–93 (1955).

Rose, C. and Bell, B.: Predicting longevity (Heath Lexington Books, Lexington 1971).

Rosenmayr, L.: Soziologie des Alters. In: *R. König* (Ed.): Hdbch. d. emp. Sozialforsch. *2:* 306–357 (Enke, Stuttgart 1969).

Rosow, I.: The social context of the aging self. Gerontologist *13:* 82–87 (1973).

**Rudinger, G.:* Intelligenz im Alter; phil. Diss. Bonn (1971a).

**Rudinger, G.:* Determinanten der intellektuellen Leistung im höheren Alter. actuelle gerontologie *1:* 731–737 (1971b).

**Rudinger, G.:* Zur Struktur der intellektuellen Leistungsfähigkeit im höheren Alter. actuelle gerontologie *1:* 135–140 (1971c).

**Rudinger, G.:* Determinanten der intellektuellen Leistung. Arch. Psychol. *124:* 27–38 (1972a).

Rudinger, G.: Methoden der Längsschnittforschung. I. Z. Geront. *5:* 397–424 (1972b).

**Rudinger, G.:* Intellektuelle Leistung im Alter. Z. präklin. Geriatrie *2:* 65–68 (1972c).

**Rudinger, G.:* The application of time- and cross-sequential strategies on intelligence data of the Bonn Longitudinal Study. Paper read at 2nd Meet. Int. Soc. for Study of Behavioral Development (Ann Arbor 1973a).

**Rudinger, G.:* Intellectual de-differentiation and deficit with age – artifacts? Gerontologia *19:* 253–262 (1973b).

Rudinger, G.: Eine Querschnittuntersuchung im Altersbereich 20–90 Jahre. Z. Geront. *7:* 323–333 (1974).

**Rudinger, G.:* Untersuchungen zur Methodik von Auswertung und Interpretation der Beziehungen von Persönlichkeit und Leistung im höheren Alter. Schlußbericht A2–4496 für das Landesamt für Forschung des Landes NRW (Westdeutscher Verlag, Opladen, im Druck, 1975).

**Rudinger, G. und Erlemeier, N.:* Längsschnittuntersuchungen zum Problem des Zusammenhanges von Persönlichkeit und Leistung im höheren Lebensalter, vol. 3, pp. 240–248 (Deutsche Gesellschaft für Gerontologie, Darmstadt 1970).

**Rudinger, G. und Feger, H.:* Die Beurteilung formaler Verhaltensmerkmale durch Rating-Skalen: eine Generalisierbarkeitsstudie. Z. EntwPsychol. pädag. Psychol. *2:* 96–112 (1970).

**Rudinger, G. u. Schmitz-Scherzer, R.:* Alternsprozesse (Kohlhammer, Stgt., im Druck, 1976).

Savage, R. D. and Britton, P. G.: The factorial structure of the WAIS in an aged sample. J. Geront *23:* 183–184 (1968).

Savage, R. D.; Britton, P. G.; Bolton, N., and Hall, E. H.: Intellectual functioning in the aged (Methuen, London 1973).

Schaie, K. W.: Rigidity-flexibility and intelligence. Psychol. Monogr. *72:* 462–488 (1958).

Schaie, K. W.: A general model for the study of developmental problems. Psychol. Bull. *64:* 92–107 (1965).

Schaie, K. W.: A reinterpretation of age related changes in cognitive structure and functioning; in *Goulet and Baltes* Life-span developmental psychology: research and theory (Academic Press, New York 1970).

Schaie, K. W.: Limitations on generalizability of growth curves of intelligence. A reanalysis of data from the Harvard Study. Hum. Dev. *15:* 141–152 (1972a).

Schaie, K. W.: Can the longitudinal method be applied to psychological studies of human development? in *Moenks, Hartup and de Wit* Determinants of behavioural development, pp. 3–22 (Academic Press, New York 1972b).

Schaie, K. W.: Methodological problems in the descriptive developmental research on adulthood and aging; in *Nesselroade and Reese* Life-span developmental psychology: methodological issues (Academic Press, New York 1973).

Schaie, K. W. and Baltes, P. B.: Comments on Buss' theories of sequential strategies in developmental research: is description or explanation of developmental change at stake? Draft (1975).

Schaie, K. W. and Gribbin, K.: Adult development and aging. A. Rev. Psychol. *26:* 65–96 (1975).

Schaie, K. W. und Gribbin, K.: Umwelteinflüsse auf die Persönlichkeitsentwicklung im Erwachsenenalter. Z. EntwPsychol. pädag. Psychol. *8* (im Druck, 1976).

Schaie, K. W.; Labouvie, G. V., and Buech, B. U.: Generational and cohort-specific differences in adult cognitive functioning: a fourteen-year study of independent samples. Devl Psychol. *9:* 151–166 (1973).

Schaie, K. W. and Labouvie-Vief, G. V.: Generational versus ontogenetic components of change in adult cognitive behavior: a fourteen-year cross-sequential study. Devl Psychol. *10:* 305–320 (1974).

Schaie, K. W. and Strother, C. R.: A cross-sequentional study of age changes in cognitive behavior. Psychol. Bull. *70:* 671–680 (1968a).

Schaie, K. W. and Strother, C. R.: The effects of time- and cohort differences on the interpretation of age changes in cognitive behavior. Multivar. Behav. Res. *3:* 259–294 (1968b).

Schick, F. V.; Dahlhaus, C.; Hartnack, C. und Osthoff, I.: Faktorenanalytische Untersuchungen zur Methodenabhängigkeit bei Faktorenmustern von Wechsler-Intelligenztests; unveröffentlichte Vorexamensarbeit Bonn (1972).

Schmid, M.: Wesen und Aufgabe der Gerontologie in medizingeschichtlicher Sicht. Ber. Symp. Dt. Ges. Gerontologie, Nürnberg 1973 (Banaschewski, München).

**Schmitz-Scherzer, R.:* Freizeit und Alter; phil. Diss. Bonn (1969).

Schmitz-Scherzer, R.: Freizeit-Andragogik als Instrument psychologischer Rehabilitation; in *Störmer* Geroprophylaxe, Infektions- und Herzkrankheiten, Rehabilitation und Sozialstatus im Alter, pp. 284–289 (Steinkopff, Darmstadt 1970).

Schmitz-Scherzer, R.: Freizeitverhalten und sozialer Kontext. Z. Sozialpsychol. *3:* 116–125 (1972).

Schmitz-Scherzer, R.: Freizeit im Alter (Deutsche Gesellschaft für Freizeit, Düsseldorf 1973).

Schmitz-Scherzer, R.: Freizeit (Akademische Verlagsgesellschaft, Frankfurt 1974a).

Schmitz-Scherzer, R.: Sozialpsychologie der Freizeit (Kohlhammer, Stuttgart 1974b).

**Schmitz-Scherzer, R.:* Veränderungen des Freizeitverhaltens. actuelle gerontologie *5:* 103–106 (1975a).

**Schmitz-Scherzer, R.:* Konstanz und Variabilität im Alltagsverhalten Älterer – eine Längsschnittanalyse über 5 Jahre. Z. Geront. *8* (im Druck, 1975b).

*Schmitz-Scherzer, R.: Probleme der psychischen Entwicklung im Alter; phil. Habilitationsschrift Bonn (1975c).

*Schmitz-Scherzer, R. und Angleitner, A.: Intellektuelle Leistungsfähigkeit im mittleren und höheren Erwachsenenalter aus persönlichkeits- und entwicklungspsychologischer Sicht; in *Lehr und Weinert* Entwicklung und Persönlichkeit (Kohlhammer, Suttgart 1975).

*Schmitz-Scherzer, R. und Lehr, U.: Gesundheitliches Wohlbefinden und psychischer Alternsprozeß. Medizin des alternden Menschen *6:* 175–178 (1971).

*Schmitz-Scherzer, R.; Renner, M. und Olbrich, E.: Freizeit und Alter; in *Schubert* Herz und Atmungsorgane im Alter, Psychologie und Soziologie in der Gerontologie, pp. 252–260 (Steinkopff, Darmstadt 1968).

*Schmitz-Scherzer, R. and Stroedel, I.: Age dependencies of leisure activities. Hum. Dev. *14:* 47–50 (1971).

Schmitz-Scherzer, R.; Thomae, H.; Angleitner, A.; Bierhoff, H. W; Grombach, H.; Rudinger, G. und Steffens K. H.: Altenhilfe 2. Berichte der Landesregierung von NRW, pp. 81–105 (Ministerium für Arbeit und Gesundheit, Düsseldorf 1974).

*Schneider, H.: Untersuchung zum Zusammenhang zwischen Reaktionszeit und Auffassungssicherheit; unveröffentlichte psychologische Vorexamensarbeit Bonn (1967).

Schoenfeldt, L. F.: Life history subgroups on moderators in the prediction of intellectual change; in *Jarvik et al.* Intellectual functioning in adults (Springer, New York 1973).

Schooler, K. K.: The relationship between social interaction and morale of the elderly as a function of environmental characteristics. Gerontologist *9:* 25–29 (1969).

*Schreiner, M.: Zur zukunftsbezogenen Zeitperspektive älterer Menschen; phil. Diss. Bonn (1969).

*Schreiner, M.: Zur zukunftsbezogenen Zeitperspektive älterer Menschen. Z. EntwPsychol. pädag. Psychol. *2:* 28 (1970a).

*Schreiner, M.: Inhaltliche Aspekte der zukunftsbezogenen Zeitperspektive bei älteren Menschen. Z. EntwPsychol. pädag. Psychol. *2:* 149 (1970b).

*Schreiner, M.: Gegenwärtige Lebenssituation und Zukunftsgedanken älterer Menschen. Z. Geront. *3:* 272–282 (1970c).

*Schreiner, M.: Dimensionen der Gegenwarts- und Zukunftsorientierung bei älteren Menschen (Längsschnittstudie). actuelle gerontologie *12:* 715–719 (1971a).

*Schreiner, M.: Zum Erleben der gegenwärtigen und zukünftigen Lebenssituation älterer Menschen. Arch. Psychol. *123:* 268–284 (1971b).

*Schreiner, M.; Rudinger, G. und Schmitz-Scherzer, R.: Veränderungen der psychomotorischen Leistungsfähigkeit im höheren Erwachsenenalter. actuelle gerontologie *1:* 141–147 (1971).

Schubert, R.: Verschiedene Formen des Alterns. In: *Schubert, R.* (Ed.): Flexibilität der Altergrenze. pp. 1–3 (Sternkopff, Darmstadt 1969).

Schwarz, K.: Voraussichtliche Entwicklung der Zahl älterer Menschen und ihrer Lebenserwartung; in *Schubert und Störmer* Schwerpunkte in der Geriatrie, vol. 3, pp. 17–19 (Werk Verlag, München-Gräfelfing 1974).

Secord, P. F. and Backman, C.: Social psychology (McGraw-Hill, New York 1964).

Selugga, A.: Vergleichsuntersuchung zur Reaktionsgeschwindigkeit zehnjähriger Jungen und Mädchen; unveröffentlichte psychologische Vorexamensarbeit Bonn (1969).

Shang Wang, H. and Busse, E. W.: Brain impairment and longevity; in *Palmore* Normal aging, pp. 263–268 (Duke University Press, Durham 1974).

Shelton, F. C. and Kogan, N.: Images of 'old people' and 'people in general' in an older sample. J. genet. Psychol. *100:* 3–21 (1962).

*Simons, H.; Mehler, D. und Erlemeier, N.: Aspekte der psychologischen Anpassung im höheren Lebensalter, vol. 1, pp. 215–223 (Deutsche Gesellschaft für Gerontologie, Darmstadt 1968).

Singer, M. T.: Personality measurements in the aged; in *Birren et al.* Human aging, pp. 217–249 (National Institute of Mental Health, Bethesda 1963); German in *Thomae und Lehr* Altern – Probleme und Tatsachen, pp. 171–202 (Akademische Verlagsgesellschaft, Frankfurt 1968).

Sixtl, F.: Ein Verfahren zur Rotation von Faktorenladungen nach einem vorgegebenen Kriterium. Arch. Psychol. *116:* 92–97 (1964).

Spieth, W.: Cardiovascular health status, age, and psychological performance. J. Geront. *19:*

Stern, E.: Der Mensch in der zweiten Lebenshälfte. (Rascher, Zürich 1955).

Stone, J. L. and Norris, A. H.: Activities and attitudes of participants in the Baltimore longitudinal study. J. Geront. *21:* 575–580 (1966).

Streib, G. F. and Orbach, H. L.: Aging; in *Lazarsfeld et al.* The uses of sociology, pp. 612–640 (Basic Books, New York 1967).

Terman, L. M. and Oden, M. H.: The gifted group at mid-life (University Press, Stanford 1959).

**Theissen, C.:* Untersuchungen zum Selbstbild älterer Menschen; phil. Diss. Bonn (1970a).

**Theissen, C.:* Das Selbstbild des Alters als Spiegelbild des Altersbildes der Gesellschaft. Ber. Kongr. Dt. Ges. Psychologie, pp. 239–246 (Steinkopff, Darmstadt 1970b).

Thomae, H.: Objective socialization variables in personality development. Hum. Dev. *8:* 87–116 (1965).

**Thomae, H.:* Psychische und soziale Aspekte des Alterns. Z. Geront. *1:* 43–55 (1968a).

Thomae, H.: Das Individuum und seine Welt. Eine Persönlichkeitstheorie (Hogrefe, Göttingen 1968b).

**Thomae, H.:* Persönlichkeit und Alter. Ber. Kongr. Dt. Ges. Gerontologie, Nürnberg 1967, pp. 191–203 (Steinkopff, Darmstadt 1968c).

Thomae, H.: Zur Entwicklungs- und Sozialpsychologie des alternden Menschen; in *Thomae und Lehr* Altern – Probleme und Tatsachen, pp. 3–17 (Akademische Verlagsgesellschaft, Frankfurt 1968d).

**Thomae, H.:* Altern als psychologisches Problem; in *Irle* Ber. 26. Kongr. Dt. Ges. Psychologie, Tübingen 1958, pp. 22–36 (Hogrefe, Göttingen 1969).

Thomae, H.: Theory of aging and cognitive theory of personality. Hum. Dev. *13:* 1–16 (1970).

Thomae, H.: Beobachtung und Beurteilung von Kindern und Jugendlichen; 10. Aufl. (Karger, Basel 1971a).

Thomae, H.: Die Bedeutung einer kognitiven Persönlichkeitstheorie für die Theorie des Alterns. Z. Geront. *4:* 8–18 (1971b).

Thomae, H.: Soziale Schichten als Sozialisationsvariablen; in *Graumann* Handbuch der Psychologie, vol. 7, pp. 748ff. (Hogrefe, Göttingen 1972).

Thomae, H.: Anpassungsprobleme im höheren Alter – aus psychologischer Sicht. actuelle gerontologie *4:* 647–656 (1974a).

Thomae, H.: Introduction; in *Thomae and Endo* The adolescent and his environment. Contributions to an ecology of teen-age behavior, pp. 1–11 (Karger, Basel 1974b).

Thomae, H. und Lehr, U.: Altern – Probleme und Tatsachen (Akademische Verlagsgesellschaft, Frankfurt 1968).

**Thomae, H.; Angleitner, A.; Grombach, H. und Schmitz-Scherzer, R.:* Determinanten und Varianten des Alternsprozesses. Ein Bericht über die Bonner gerontologische Längsschnittstudie. actuelle gerontologie *3:* 359–377 (1973).

Thomae, H. und Lehr, U.: Berufliche Leistungsfähigkeit im mittleren und höheren Erwachsenenalter (Schwartz, Göttingen 1973).

*_Thomae, H. und Simons, H.:_ Reaktionen auf Belastungssituationen im höheren Alter. Z. exp. angew. Psychol. _14:_ 290–312 (1967).

Thomlinson, R.: Population dynamics, causes and consequences of world demographic change (Random House, New York 1965).

*_Tismer, K. G.:_ Untersuchungen zur Lebensthematik älterer Menschen; phil. Diss. Bonn (1969).

*_Tismer, K. G.:_ Zur sozialen Lebensthematik im höheren Erwachsenenalter. Ber. 3. Kongr. Dt. Ges. Gerontologie, pp. 89–95 (Steinkopff, Darmstadt 1970).

*_Tismer, K. G.:_ Leistungsfähigkeit in der Sicht älterer Menschen. actuelle gerontologie _1:_ 153–160 (1971).

Tuckman, J. and Lorge, I.: Old people's appraisal of adjustment over the life-span. J. Personality _22:_ 417–422 (1954).

Tuddenham, L. D.; Blumenkrantz, J., and Wilkin, W. R.: Age changes on ACCT: a longitudinal study of average adults. J. consult. Psychol. _32:_ 659–663 (1968).

Tulkin, S. R. and Konner, M. J.: Alternative conceptions of intellectual functioning. Hum. Dev. _16:_ 33–52 (1973).

Ueberla, K.: Faktorenanalyse (Springer, Berlin 1968).

Van den Daele, L. D.: Qualitative models in developmental analysis. Dev. Psychol. _1:_ 303–310 (1969).

Vernon, P. E.: The variation of intelligence with occupation, age, and locality. Br. J. Psychol. _1:_ 57–63 (1947).

Vischer, A. L.: Seelische Wandlungen beim alternden Menschen (Schwabe, Basel 1949).

Wagner, E. E.: Differences beetween old and young executives on objective psychological test variables. J. Geront. _15:_ 296–299 (1960).

Wall, D. and Williams, H. L.: Longitudinal studies and the social sciences (Heinemann, London 1970).

Wechsler, D.: Die Messung der Intelligenz Erwachsener; 3. Aufl. (Huber, Bern 1964).

Weinstock, C. and Bennett, R.: The relation between social isolation and related cognitive skills of a catholic and Jewish home for the aged. Proc. 8th Int. Congr. on Gerontology, Washington 1969, vol. 2, p. 98 (International Gerontological Society, Washington 1969).

Welford, A. T.: Psychomotor performance; in _Birren_ Handbook of aging and the individual (University of Chicago Press, Chicago 1959, 1967).

Welford, A. T.: Industrial work for older people: some British studies. Gerontologist _6:_ 4–9 (1966).

Welford, A. T. and Birren, J. E.: Behavior, aging, and the nervous system (Thomas, Springfield 1965).

Weston, H. C.: The effect of age and illumination upon visual performance with close sights. Br. J. Ophthal. _32:_ (1948).

Wiendieck, G.: Zur psychosozialen Bedingtheit des Alterssuicids. actuelle gerontologie _3:_ 271–274 (1973).

Wilcoxon, F.: Individual comparisons by ranking tests. Biometrics _1:_ 80–82 (1945).

*_Wildermuth, G.:_ Reaktionsschnelligkeit und psychophysische Belastbarkeit im höheren Lebensalter; unveröffentlichte psychologische Vorexamensarbeit Bonn (1971).

Wiley, D. E. and Wiley, J. A.: An estimation of measurement error in panel data; in _Blalock_ Causal models in the social sciences (Macmillan, London 1971).

Wilkie, F. and Eisdorfer, C.: Terminal changes in intelligence. Gerontologist _12:_ 67–72 (1972).

Wilkie, F. L. and Eisdorfer, C.: Systemic disease and behavioral correlates; in _Jarvik, Eisdorfer and Blum_ Intellectual functioning in adults: psychological and biological influences, pp. 83–94 (Springer, New York 1973).

Williams, R. H. and Wirths, C. G.: Lives through the years. (Wiley, New York 1965).

Winer, B.: Statistical principles in experimental design; 2nd ed. (McGraw-Hill, New York 1971).

Wohlwill, J. F.: Methodology and research strategy in the study of developmental change; in *Goulet and Baltes* Life-span developmental psychology, pp. 150–190 (Academic Press, New York 1970).

Yarrow, L. J. and Bayley, N.: Symposium on personality consistency and change. Vita hum. 7: 65–146 (1964).

Youmans, E. G. and Yarrow, M. R.: Twelve year follow-up study of healthy older men: social psychological data. Proc. 8th Int Congr. on Gerontology, p. 84 (International Gerontological Society, Washington 1969).

Zimmermann, M. E.: Untersuchung über Veränderungen der psychischen Leistungsfähigkeit bei cerebraler Durchblutungsstörung; unveröffentlichte psychologische Vorexamensarbeit Bonn (1971).